Disorders of Neonatal Glycemia

David H. Adamkin • William W. Hay, Jr.
Editors

Disorders of Neonatal Glycemia

Neonatal Glucose Extremes, Hypoglycemia and Hyperglycemia

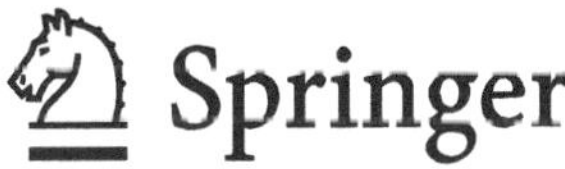

Editors
David H. Adamkin
Division of Neonatal Medicine
University of Louisville
Louisville, Kentucky, USA

William W. Hay, Jr.
University of Colorado
Denver, CO, USA

ISBN 978-3-032-29093-9 ISBN 978-3-032-29094-6 (eBook)
https://doi.org/10.1007/978-3-032-29094-6

This Springer imprint is published by the registered company Springer Nature Switzerland AG
The registered company address is: Gewerbestrasse 11, 6330 Cham, Switzerland

I dedicate this book to my wife, Carol, my best friend and academic collaborator my whole career.

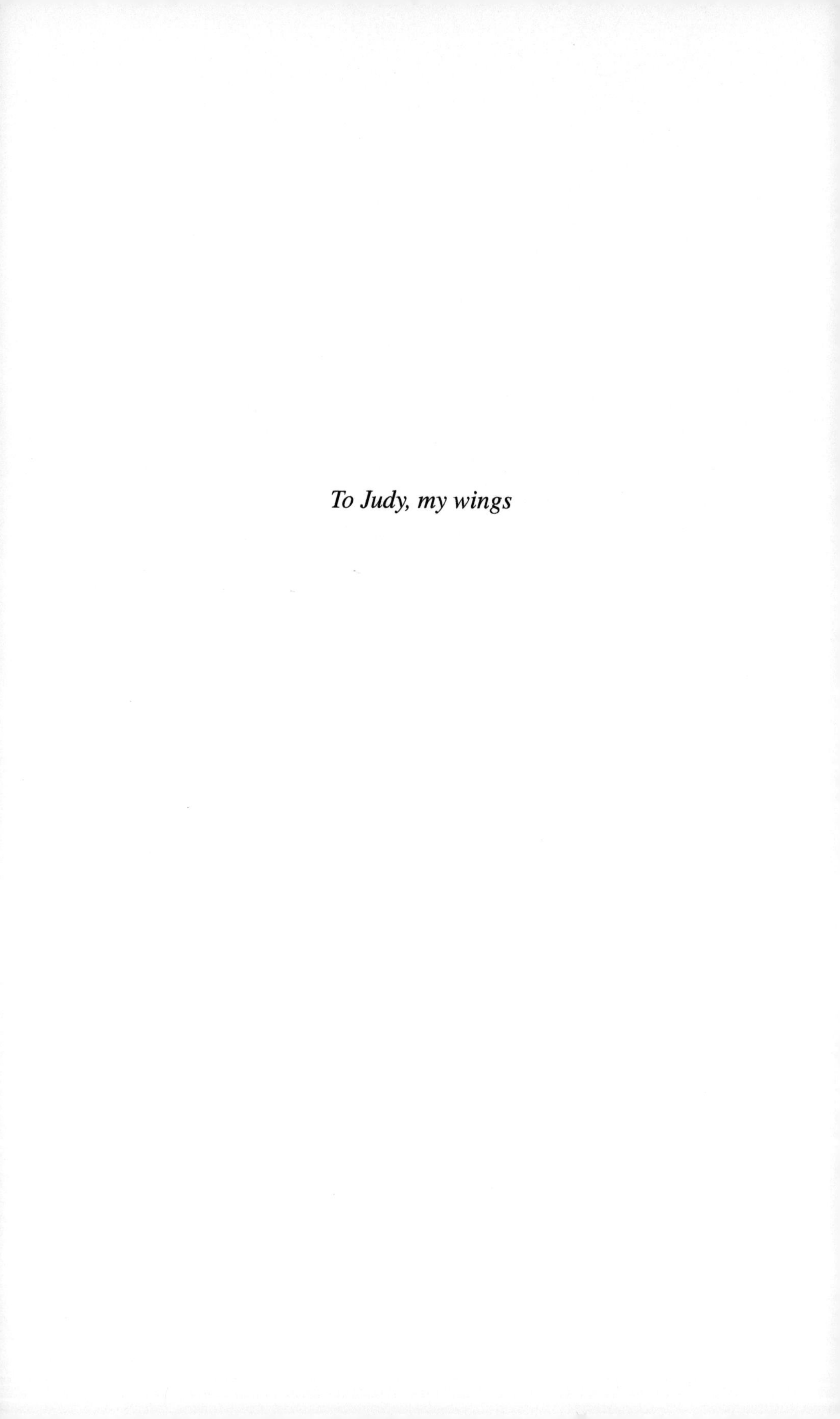

To Judy, my wings

Contents

Contributors

David H. Adamkin Division of Neonatal Medicine, University of Louisville, Louisville, Kentucky, USA

Jane Alsweiler Department of Paediatrics: Child and Youth Health, School of Medicine, University of Auckland, Auckland, New Zealand

Kristin Harrison Ginsberg Department of Paediatrics: Child and Youth Health, School of Medicine, University of Auckland, Auckland, New Zealand

Jane Harding Liggins Institute, University of Auckland, Auckland, New Zealand

William W. Hay, Jr. University of Colorado, Denver, CO, USA

Part I
Neonatal Glucose Extremes

Chapter 1
Introduction

David H. Adamkin and William W. Hay, Jr.

Newborn infants, especially those born preterm, frequently experience extremes of glucose metabolism and plasma concentrations [1]. These extremes, hypoglycemia and hyperglycemia, each have unique and pathological consequences. This is particularly true for the brain and the potentially adverse impacts of hypoglycemia and hyperglycemia particularly with relatively prolonged duration.

But why focus primarily on glucose concentrations in the circulation? We cannot easily measure brain blood flow, yet many conditions in preterm infants reduce circulation and thus glucose delivery to the brain. We also cannot measure brain glucose uptake easily, yet that is the best measure of sufficient or insufficient glucose supply to the brain. Brain glucose uptake and metabolism are directly related to plasma glucose concentration in the normal plasma glucose concentration range and reach maximum rates at the higher end of the normal range. Unfortunately, the correlation between plasma glucose concentration and the consequences of insufficient or excess brain glucose supply and metabolism are poor, which has created misunderstanding and confusion [2].

D. H. Adamkin (✉)
Division of Neonatal Medicine, University of Louisville, Louisville, Kentucky, USA
e-mail: david.adamkin@louisville.edu

W. W. Hay, Jr.
University of Colorado, Denver, CO, USA
e-mail: bill.hay@ucdenver.edu

D. H. Adamkin, W. W. Hay, Jr. (eds.), *Disorders of Neonatal Glycemia*,
https://doi.org/10.1007/978-3-032-29094-6_1

Hypoglycemia

Severe and prolonged hypoglycemia has long been recognized for its detrimental effects on the neonatal brain. Glucose supply to the brain is fundamental, because the brain uses glucose as its primary substrate for oxidative metabolism. The brain uses about 20 times more glucose than muscle or fat does, and neonates have a relatively large brain to body weight ratio (12%) compared to that in adults (2%). This produces a threefold higher body weight-specific glucose utilization rate in the neonate, about 6 mg/min/kg vs. the adult at about 2 mg/min/kg. Ninety percent of whole-body glucose utilization occurs in the neonatal brain, which makes the brain particularly susceptible to glucose deprivation, reduced oxidative glucose metabolism, and disruption of normal neural function. These adverse effects may lead to seizures, impaired neurological development, mental retardation, and even death [3]. If glucose deprivation to the brain is prolonged, permanent neuronal damage can occur. There still is lack of certainty about how low plasma glucose needs to be and for how long to damage the brain, and whether it is just very low concentrations in the plasma or intermittently low and highly variable concentrations affecting brain glucose supply that are the most damaging to developing neurons [4]. Clinical signs of hypoglycemia may often be indistinguishable from other clinical disorders and are poorly predictive of neurological damage. Despite these limitations in making hard and fast lower limits for neonatal glucose concentrations, over many years, this problem has not changed except for arbitrary increases in lower limits of "normal" neonatal glucose concentrations. This has been done without evidence that outcomes from preventing or treating glucose concentrations lower than such lower limits were improved or even affected (Fig. 1.1).

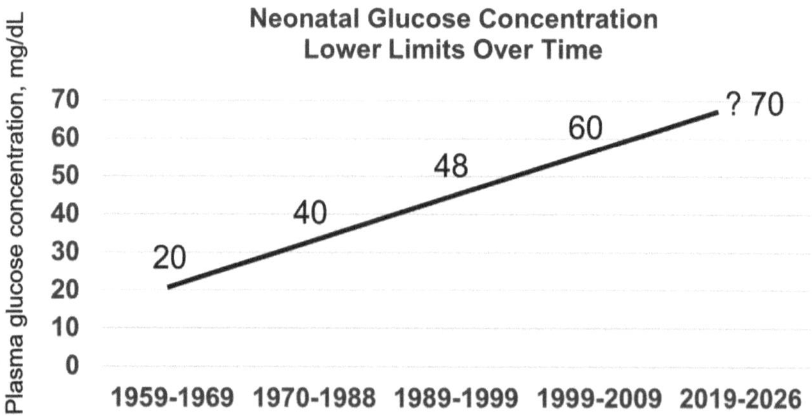

Fig. 1.1 Arbitrary increase over the past 50+ years in the estimated lower limit of normal neonatal plasma glucose concentrations. (Adapted from Cornblath (2000) and Hay (2009, 2019), as presented at the Hot Topics meeting)

Why does neonatal hypoglycemia continue to be so controversial and important? Primarily because low circulating glucose concentrations are not a good measure of brain glucose metabolism, nor are they a good measure of neuronal function, neuronal viability, irreparable neuronal damage, or longer term potentially adverse neurodevelopmental outcomes. There still is no clear and evidence-based definition of "clinically significant" (damaging) neonatal hypoglycemia, nor the duration of any low glucose concentration on adverse outcomes. Hypoglycemia is common, and only observational "evidence" (not data from controlled, prospective investigations) documents "apparent neurological injury" with severe hypoglycemia in human neonates.

Symptomatic hypoglycemic infants, primarily those with severe, protracted, and recurrent neurological conditions such as seizures and coma, with plasma glucose concentrations of zero to 1.1–1.4 mmolL (20–25 mg/dL) for several hours or more, have a poorer prognosis These are associated with abnormalities ranging from learning disabilities to cerebral palsy and persistent or recurrent seizure disorders, as well as mental retardation of varying degrees [5].

Hyperglycemia

Hyperglycemia also has significantly adverse impact on neuronal function and development [6, 7]. There are no demonstrable clinical signs of hyperglycemia so it must be measured to know it is present. Because of the lack of clinical manifestations, many have considered hyperglycemia, especially when transient and occurring primarily right after birth for short durations, of little clinical significance. Many studies in animal models and clinical studies in human infants, however, have shown adverse effects of acute and long-term hyperglycemia on developing neurons that have lasting adverse impact on later life, resulting in neurodisability and cognitive deficits. Furthermore, excess glucose in many cells produces reactive oxygen species that can damage local cellular components and leak into the circulation and cause cellular damage throughout the body. It remains unclear whether modest and transient increased glucose concentrations lead to permanent adverse outcomes, but the highest glucose concentrations, those greater than 270 mg/dL (>15 mmol/L), have been associated with adverse neurodevelopmental outcomes [8], and longer durations of hyperglycemia have been strongly associated with many adverse conditions and even death [9].

The aim of this book is to review recent literature, including primary research and recent reviews, to examine what we understand about these extremes of plasma glucose concentrations in newborn infants. This book will not review the mostly genetic causes of hyper- and hypoglycemia as those are well covered in recent textbooks. The chapters are comprehensive reviews. They do include reports of meta-analyses or systematic reviews from publications by other authors, as well as primary data in research publications. The chapters, however, are only intended to be interpretations of the data in the literature by the authors of this book.

References

1. Sunehag AL, Haymond MW. Glucose extremes in newborn infants. Clin Perinatol. 2002;29:245–60.
2. Hay WW Jr. Recent observations on the regulation of fetal metabolism by glucose. J Physiol. 2006;572:17–24.
3. Siesjo BK. Hypoglycemia, brain metabolism, and brain damage. Diabetes Metab Rev. 1988;4:113–44.
4. Stanley CA, Caplin N. Pathophysiology of hypoglycemia. In: Polin R, Abman S, Fox W, editors. Fetal and neonatal physiology. 3rd ed. Philadelphia: WB Saunders; 2003.
5. Rozance PJ, Hay WW. Hypoglycemia in newborn infants: features associated with adverse outcomes. Biol Neonate. 2006;90:74–86.
6. Rozance PJ, Hay WW Jr. Neonatal hyperglycemia. NeoReviews. 2010;11:e632.
7. Hay WW Jr, Rozance PJ. Neonatal hyperglycemia-causes, treatments, and cautions. J Pediatr. 2018;200:6–8.
8. Minamitani Y, Nakajima K, Namba F. Association of hyperglycemia in extremely preterm infants with neurodevelopmental outcomes at 18 months of corrected age. J Perinatol. 2025;45:1370–6.
9. Stensvold HJ, Strommen K, Lang AM, Abrahamsen TG, Steen EK, Pripp AH, Ronnestad AE. Early enhance parenteral nutrition, hyperglycemia, and death among extremely low-birth-weight infants. JAMA Pediatr. 2015;169:1003–10.

Part II
Normal Fetal and Neonatal Glucose Metabolism

Chapter 2
Normal Fetal Glucose Metabolism

William W. Hay, Jr.

Placental Glucose Uptake, Metabolism, and Transfer to the Fetus

A large variety of experiments have defined how glucose is normally transferred from the maternal plasma to the fetus. Most of the in vivo studies have used the pregnant sheep as a model, while in situ perfused human placentas and in vitro isolated syncytiotrophoblasts also have been used. More detailed reviews describe the many processes involved in maternal, placental, and fetal glucose metabolism [1–4].

Under normal conditions, the placenta transfers all the glucose used by the fetus from the maternal plasma according to the maternal to fetal plasma glucose concentration gradient. The placenta not only transfers glucose to the fetus but consumes glucose for its own metabolism. Placental glucose uptake and transfer to the fetus are mediated by independent, facilitative transporter proteins on both the maternal-facing microvillus (MVM) and fetal-facing basal membranes (BMs) of the syncytiotrophoblasts [5, 6]. The predominant placental glucose transporters are GLUT1 and GLUT3. GLUT4 has been found in the syncytiotrophoblasts [6], but there is no evidence that insulin mediates placental glucose transport to the fetus. GLUTs 8, 9a, 9b, 10, and 12 have been found in late gestation human placentas, and although at least GLUTs 8, 9a, and 9b appear decreased with placental and fetal growth restriction, the roles of these transporters in placental glucose transport are not defined [7, 8].

GLUT1 accounts for most of glucose transport throughout gestation. It is expressed throughout the placenta, particularly in the syncytiotrophoblasts. It is acutely upregulated by hypoxia and hyperglycemia, but downregulated by low maternal and fetal glucose concentrations, diminishing glucose transport [9–11]. GLUT3 also determines placental glucose transport to the fetus, primarily in early

W. W. Hay, Jr. (✉)
University of Colorado, Denver, CO, USA
e-mail: bill.hay@ucdenver.edu

D. H. Adamkin, W. W. Hay, Jr. (eds.), *Disorders of Neonatal Glycemia*,
https://doi.org/10.1007/978-3-032-29094-6_2

gestation. Reduced GLUT3 in the first half of gestation results in diminished fetal growth, impaired placental glucose transport and net fetal glucose uptake, lower fetal glucose concentrations, and reduced fetal pancreatic growth and function including reduced insulin and glucagon concentrations [12–17]. GLUT3 has a five-fold greater affinity and transport capacity for glucose compared with GLUT1. Its primary location is on the MVM membrane and close to trophoblast mitochondria, which could support placental glucose consumption at low glucose concentrations [14]. GLUT3 is upregulated under hypoxia conditions, which might enhance placental glucose consumption but reduce glucose supply to the fetus, thereby contributing to fetal growth restriction [16–18]. GLUT1 and GLUT3 are downregulated by glucocorticoids. This might account for how maternal stress can lead to placental insufficiency and IUGR [19].

Kinetics of Glucose Uptake, Metabolism, and Transport by the Placenta

The uptake, consumption, and transfer of glucose by the placenta are directly related to the maternal plasma glucose concentration according to saturation kinetics (Fig. 2.1a) [20–22]. But placental-to-fetal glucose transfer also is regulated by the fetal glucose concentration and thus the maternal-to-fetal glucose concentration gradient, regardless of the maternal glucose concentration (Fig. 2.1b), indicating that the fetal side of the placenta is markedly more permeable to glucose than the maternal side. Maternal glucose concentration determines glucose entry into the

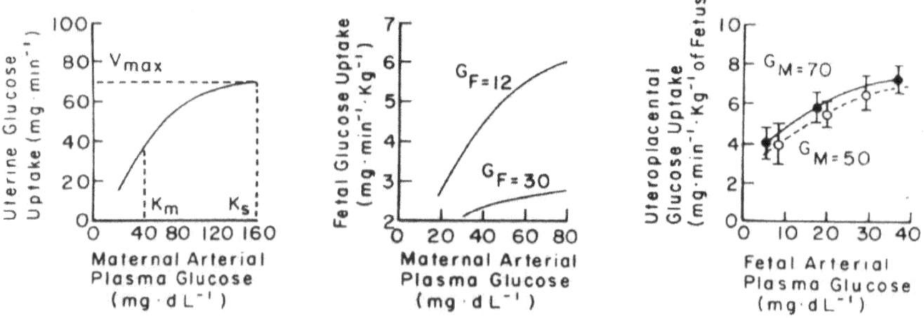

Fig. 2.1 Data from experiments in pregnant sheep using direct intravenous glucose infusions into the maternal or the fetal circulation. Uterine glucose uptake is directly related to the maternal glucose concentration according to saturation kinetics (**a**). Fetal glucose uptake (net transfer of glucose from the placenta into the fetal circulation) is directly related to the maternal glucose concentration according to saturation kinetics but also is directly related to the maternal-fetal glucose concentration gradient (**b**). The net rate of uteroplacental glucose consumption is directly related to the fetal arterial plasma glucose much more than the maternal glucose concentration (**c**). (Reproduced from Hay [53]). (**a**). (Adapted from data in Refs. [20, 21]) (**b, c**). (Adapted from data in Refs. [21, 22])

conceptus (uteroplacenta and fetus), but fetal glucose concentrations, that can increase with glucogenesis or hypoxia or decrease with excessive insulin secretion, for example, independently regulate uteroplacental glucose consumption (Fig. 2.1c) [21, 22].

Gestational Changes in Placental Glucose Transfer

Placental glucose transport increases markedly over gestation, ~60% in sheep, directly related to placental growth, MVM and BM surface area, and the number of GLUT1 and GLUT3 glucose transporters (~twofold for GLUT1 in sheep) [11]. Glucose utilization in the fetus increases over the second half of gestation via increasing fetal mass, cellularity, and glucose metabolic rate of the fetal brain and heart; progressive development of fetal insulin secretion by the expanding mass of pancreatic islets and beta cells; and increased growth of insulin-sensitive tissues, primarily skeletal muscle and heart, but also the liver and adipose tissue. These mechanisms decrease fetal glucose concentration that increases the transplacental glucose concentration gradient, thereby accounting for the remaining 40% increase in placental glucose transport in late gestation [23–25]. Mechanisms that are responsible for the relative decrease in fetal glucose concentration include the increasing size, cellularity, and glucose metabolic rate of the fetal brain and heart; progressive development of fetal insulin secretion by the expanding mass of pancreatic islets and beta cells; and increased growth of insulin-sensitive tissues, primarily skeletal muscle and heart, but also the liver and adipose tissue.

Fetal Glucose Transporters and Glucose Utilization Rate (GUR)

All organs and cells in the fetus depend on the plasma glucose concentration for their specific rates of glucose uptake and utilization. Conditions that reduce glucose supply to the fetus and fetal circulating glucose concentrations upregulate fetal tissue glucose and cellular membrane transporter expression and the capacity for glucose utilization to maintain fetal metabolism and growth. Conditions that provide excess glucose reduce glucose transporter expression in the fetus, which limits fetal tissue and cellular glucose uptake and utilization and the directly related capacity for overgrowth and excess adiposity [9, 26–28]. GUR has not been measured in the human fetus, but in near-term fetal sheep it is about 5–7 mg/min/kg [28], similar to that in term human newborn infants [29]. GUR is higher at mid-gestation in fetal sheep when fetal growth, protein turnover, and fractional protein synthetic rates are about twice those closer to term [25].

Kinetics of Fetal Glucose Utilization

Glucose utilization rates have not been measured in human fetuses, especially over the second half of gestation, but estimates from fetal sheep and from normal term human newborn infants using stable isotope measurements indicate rates of 2–3 mg/min/kg at term, and two to threefold higher at mid-gestation. In preterm humans, and thus perhaps the near term human fetus, doubling or even tripling of GUR from basal is possible [30]. Fetal GUR varies directly with maternal arterial plasma glucose concentration but can be variable when increased entry of glucose into the fetus from higher maternal glucose concentrations increases fetal glucose concentration and GUR. Insulin secretion also increases under such conditions, which, in turn, acts independently to augment fetal GUR that then lowers fetal glucose concentrations. This would in turn increase the maternal-fetal glucose concentration gradient, driving more glucose into the fetus. GUR is limited, however, and when this occurs, fetal glucose concentrations would increase in line with increasing maternal glucose concentrations [23, 25]. Both fetal plasma glucose and insulin concentrations regulate fetal glucose utilization and oxidation, reaching a maximum rate with their combined but independent effects (Fig. 2.2). Effects of increased glucose supply to the fetus are shown in Table 2.1.

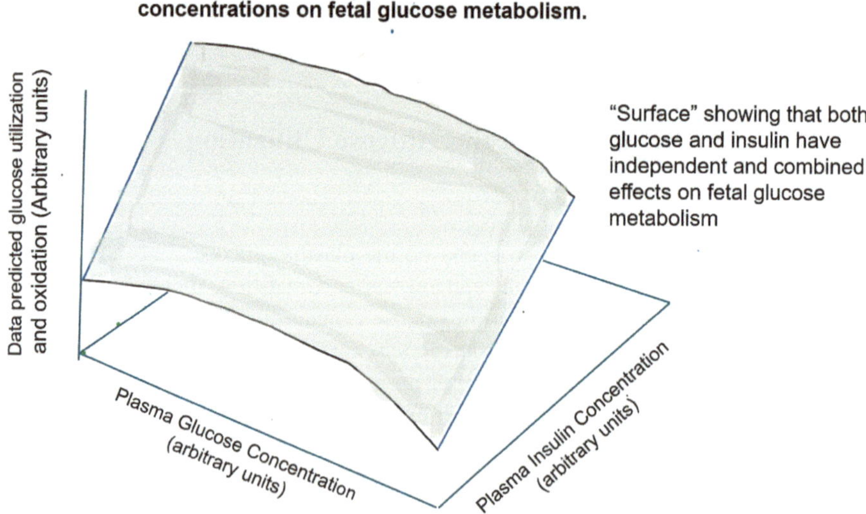

Fig. 2.2 Combined impact of glucose and insulin on fetal glucose metabolism. (Adapted from: Refs. [22, 23])

Table 2.1 Fetal metabolic and clinical responses to increased glucose supply

Short term: Mild–moderate
Increased glucose uptake from the placenta
Glucose-induced increased insulin secretion and plasma insulin concentration
Increased glucose utilization and oxidation
Increased metabolic rate (oxygen consumption)
Mildly lower arterial blood oxygen content and partial pressure
Mild hypercarbia
Increased lactate production in the fetus as well as fetal lactate utilization
Short term: Severe
Markedly lower arterial blood oxygen content and partial pressure
Increased catecholamine secretion and concentration
Lower plasma insulin concentration as suppressed by hypoxemia and catecholamines
Increased erythropoietin production
Increased metabolic rate (oxygen consumption), followed by decline with fetal demise
Metabolic acidosis
Decreased umbilical blood flow to the placenta
Fetal demise
Chronic and sustained
Decreased insulin production, secretion, and plasma concentration
Decreased insulin sensitivity in peripheral tissues, primarily skeletal muscle and heart
Increased placental glucose consumption to placental glucose transfer ratio

Modified from: Hay et al. [31]

Fetal Insulin Secretion

Glucose-stimulated fetal insulin secretion (GSIS) increases more than fivefold during the second half of gestation in fetal sheep and has been documented in third-trimester human fetuses, which is augmented in fetuses of gestational diabetic mothers [32, 33]. Fetal insulin secretion is regulated by the degree, duration, and pattern of changes in fetal plasma glucose concentration. From studies in fetal sheep, it appears that constant, high glucose concentrations over longer periods decrease GSIS [34], while acute spikes of higher glucose concentrations (pulsatile hyperglycemia) increase insulin secretion [35, 36]. In humans, this can occur with meals rich in glucose and easily digestible carbohydrates, which is common in GDMs in whom there is a strong tendency to develop increasingly exaggerated, meal-associated, "pulsatile" hyperglycemia in late gestation and associated increases in fetal and neonatal insulin secretion [37]. Thus, variability in the magnitude and the intermittent nature of fetal glucose concentration determine the magnitude of fetal GSIS, with pulsatile fetal hyperglycemia producing the largest increase in GSIS.

In contrast to variable increases in fetal plasma glucose concentration promoting GSIS, chronic fetal hypoglycemia, as occurs in IUGR fetuses with placental insufficiency or with prolonged maternal fasting, diminishes fetal pancreatic islet and β-cell mass and insulin secretion. These changes can lead to worsening fetal growth rate [38]. Increased catecholamines and cortisol from stress and hypoxia, inhibit fetal insulin secretion and action, such as with increased catecholamine and cortisol secretion in response to oxygen deprivation. These changes also decrease fetal growth rate, even at normal or increased glucose concentrations [39, 40]. Recent studies in pregnant and fetal sheep have documented that restoring oxygen (maternal oxygen inhalation) and glucose (maternal IV glucose infusion) to normal levels in the chronically IUGR fetus can return GSIS to normal [41]. This has not been studied in human pregnant women with IUGR in whom bed rest and oxygen inhalation, but not glucose supplementation, has been used to try to limit progressive IUGR.

Common but not appreciated is that IUGR fetuses from chronic placental insufficiency also can have increased basal and insulin-stimulated GUR [42, 43]. This can be augmented by maintained insulin sensitivity for glucose disposal in peripheral tissues in the IUGR fetus. In contrast, the fetal liver in chronically IUGR fetuses can become resistant to insulin suppression of glucose production, which could maintain plasma glucose concentration and GUR, particularly for the brain and heart, despite decreased glucose supply [44]. These observations from studies in fetal and neonatal sheep have not been studied in human infants with IUGR, but continued hypoglycemia, sometimes with increased basal and GSIS, have been noted and represent a challenge for neonatal prevention of recurrent hypoglycemia [45].

Glucose Carbon Contribution to Fetal Metabolic Rate

Glucose is the principal energy substrate in the fetus. Fetal glucose supply, therefore, is fundamental for supporting fetal metabolic rate or the rate of fetal oxygen consumption. It also provides energy for active transport including the cellular uptake of amino acids, net protein synthesis, and protein balance. It reduces amino acid oxidation making them more available for protein synthesis and growth. It also provides the carbon for energy stored in glycogen and fat [1]. The fetal glucose oxidation fraction (the relative amount of glucose utilization rate (GUR) that produces CO_2) is only ~0.5–0.6 [23, 46–48]. Lactate derived largely from glucose and amino acids provides the additional carbon to meet the requirements of fetal oxygen consumption.

Fetal metabolic rate is relatively fixed. Thus, excess carbon supply, such as with excess delivery of glucose into the fetus, decreases amino acid oxidation but has little effect on fetal metabolic rate. Studies in fetal sheep infused with glucose and insulin have produced a maximal acute increase of ~15% of fetal oxygen consumption [47]. Under such conditions, however, glycogen stores are maximized and in human fetuses, fat production is augmented [48]. In contrast, decreased fetal glucose supply, such as during maternal fasting, reduces fetal GUR proportionally to about 50% of normal. At that point, fetal glucose production develops to maintain GUR, initially by glycogenolysis but subsequently by gluconeogenesis [48]. There is little change in fetal oxygen consumption under such relatively acute conditions, indicating an increase in the reciprocal oxidation of glucose released from glycogen and from amino acids. Over longer periods of reduced glucose supply (e.g., >2 weeks), amino acid oxidation increasingly substitutes for glucose oxidation to maintain fetal oxygen consumption, which decreases by up to 25–30%. The utilization of amino acids for oxidation decreases fetal protein accretion rates, which limits the requirement for energy substrates to maintain protein synthesis, net protein balance, and growth [49]. As a result, growth also is limited to about the same extent.

Fetal Glucose Contribution to Glycogen Formation

Glucose contributes significantly over the second half of gestation to the formation of glycogen in the placenta and in skeletal muscle, heart, liver, lung, and brain in the fetus [2]. Glycogen in most cells within the fetus contributes glucose for local cellular metabolism. In contrast, liver glycogen is unique and essential for systemic glucose needs immediately after birth because only the liver contains sufficient glucose-6-phosphatase for the release of glucose into the circulation.

Fetal Glucogenesis

Under normal conditions [50] or even short-term (1–4 h, perhaps up to 24 h in human pregnant women) reductions in maternal and fetal glucose concentrations or placental-to-fetal glucose transfer, there is no evidence for fetal glucose production. Fetal glucose production only develops significantly after prolonged periods (several days) of decreased fetal glucose supply and sustained fetal hypoglycemia and hypoinsulinemia (Fig. 2.3) [51, 52]. This capacity for fetal glucose production in response to sustained fetal glucose deprivation develops in late-gestation, augmented by hormonal signals including decreased insulin and increased cortisol and catecholamines that activate phosphoenolpyruvate carboxykinase, the rate-limiting step for gluconeogenesis [53]. Cortisol also increases hepatic glucose-6-phosphatase, the enzyme responsible for the release of glucose from the liver into the circulation.

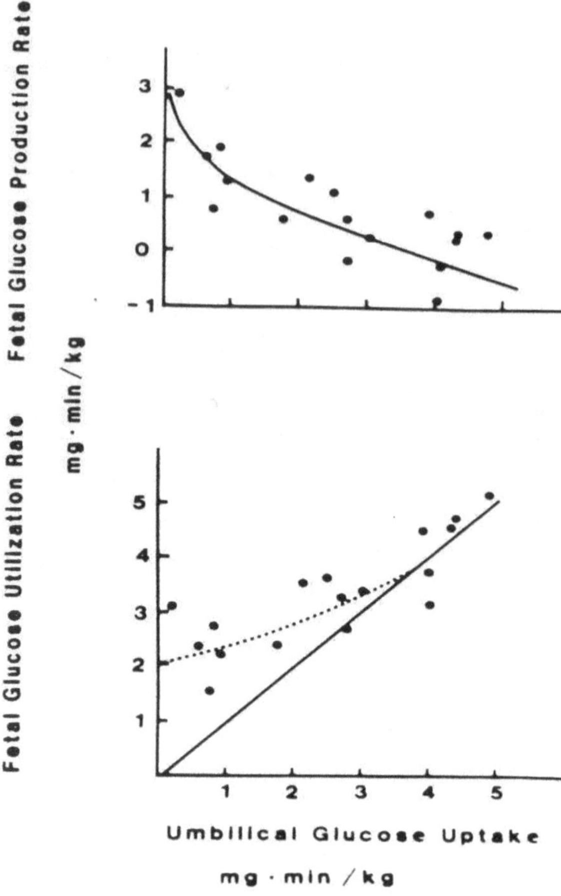

Fig. 2.3 Fetal glucose production develops in fetal sheep only after several days of maternal fasting-induced hypoglycemia. (Reproduced from Refs. [23, 48])

References

1. Hay WW Jr. Nutrient delivery and metabolism in the fetus. In: Hod M, Melamed N, Di Renzo GC, Divakar H, de Leiva-Hidalgo A, Poon LC, Yang H, Yogev Y, editors. Textbook of diabetes and pregnancy. 4th ed. Oxford: CRC Press; 2025. p. 43–56.
2. Schneider H, Reiber W, Sager R, Malek A. Asymmetrical transport of glucose across the in vitro perfused human placenta. Placenta. 2003;24:27–33.
3. Jones HN, Powell TL, Jansson T. Regulation of placental nutrient transport–a review. Placenta. 2007;28:763–74.
4. Jansson T, Wennergren M, Illsley NP. Glucose transporter protein expression in human placenta throughout gestation and in intrauterine growth retardation. J Clin Endocrinol Metab. 1993;77:1554–62.
5. Illsley NP. Glucose transporters in the human placenta. Placenta. 2000;21:14–22.
6. Ericsson A, Hamark B, Powell TL, Jansson T. Glucose transporter isoform 4 is expressed in the syncytiotrophoblast of first trimester human placenta. Hum Reprod. 2005;20:20521–2530.
7. Illsley NP, Baumann MU. Human placental glucose transport in fetoplacental growth and metabolism. Biochim Biophys Acta Mol basis Dis. 2020;1866:165359.

8. Kainulainen H, Jarvinen T, Heinonen PK. Placental glucose transporters in fetal intrauterine growth retardation and macrosomia. Gynecol Obstet Investig. 1997;44:89–92.
9. Das UG, Schroeder RE, Hay WW Jr, Devaskar SU. Time-dependent and tissue-specific effects of circulating glucose on fetal ovine glucose transporters. Am J Phys. 1999;276:R809–17.
10. Baumann MU, Zamudio S, Illsley NP. Hypoxic upregulation of glucose transporters in BeWo choriocarcinoma cells is mediated by hypoxia-inducible factor-1. Am J Physiol Cell Physiol. 2007;293:C477–85.
11. Osmond DT, Nolan CJ, King RG, Brennecke SP, Gude NM. Effects of gestational diabetes on human placental glucose uptake, transfer, and utilisation. Diabetologia. 2000;43:576–82.
12. Ehrhardt RA, Bell AW. Developmental increases in glucose transporter concentration in the sheep placenta. Am J Phys. 1997;273:R1132–41.
13. Lynch CS, Kennedy VC, Tanner AR, Ali A, Winger QA, Rozance PJ, Anthony RV. Impact of placental SLC2A3 deficiency during the first-half of gestation. Int J Mol Sci. 2022;2:12530.
14. Wooding FB, Fowden AL, Bell AW, Ehrhardt RA, Limesand SW, Hay WW. Localisation of glucose transport in the ruminant placenta: implications for sequential use of transporter isoforms. Placenta. 2005;26:626–40.
15. Janzen C, Lei MY, Cho J, Sullivan P, Shin BC, Devaskar SU. Placental glucose transporter 3 (GLUT3) is up-regulated in human pregnancies complicated by late-onset intrauterine growth restriction. Placenta. 2013;34:1072–8.
16. Zamudio S, Baumann MU, Illsley NP. Effects of chronic hypoxia in vivo on the expression of human placental glucose transporters. Placenta. 2006;27:49–55.
17. Lynch CS, Kennedy VC, Tanner AR, Ali A, Winger QA, Rozance PJ, Anthony RV. Impact of placental SLC2A3 deficiency during the first-half of gestation. Int J Mol Sci. 2022;23:12530.
18. Baumann MU, Deborde S, Illsley NP. Placental glucose transfer and fetal growth. Endocrine. 2002;19:13–22.
19. Hahn T, Barth S, Graf R, Engelmann M, Beslagic D, Reul JM, Holsboer F, Dohr G, Desoye G. Placental glucose transporter expression is regulated by glucocorticoids. J Clin Endocrinol Metab. 1999;84:1445–52.
20. Hay WW Jr, Meznarich HK. Effect of maternal glucose concentration on uteroplacental glucose consumption and transfer in pregnant sheep. Proc Soc Exp Biol Med. 1988;190:63–9.
21. Hay WW Jr, Molina RD, DiGiacomo JE, Meschia G. Model of placental glucose consumption and glucose transfer. Am J Phys. 1990;258:R569–77.
22. Hay WW Jr, DiGiacomo JE, Meznarich JK, Hirst K, Zerbe G. Effects of glucose and insulin on fetal glucose oxidation and oxygen consumption. Am J Physiol-Endo Metab. 1989;256:E704–13.
23. DiGiacomo JE, Hay WW Jr. Regulation of placental glucose transfer and consumption by fetal glucose consumption. Pediatr Res. 1989;25:429–34.
24. Michelsen TM, Holme AM, Holm MB, Roland MC, Haugen G, Powell TL, Jansson T, Henriksen T. Uteroplacental glucose uptake and fetal glucose consumption: a quantitative study in human pregnancies. J Clin Endocrinol Metab. 2019;104:873–82.
25. Molina RD, Meschia G, Battaglia FC, Hay WW Jr. Maturation of placental glucose transfer capacity in the ovine pregnancy. Am J Phys. 1991;261:R697–704.
26. Anderson MS, He J, Flowers-Ziegler J, Devaskar SU, Hay WW Jr. Effects of selective hyperglycemia and hyperinsulinemia on glucose transporters in fetal ovine skeletal muscle. Am J Phys. 2001;50:R1256–63.
27. Anderson MS, Ziegler JA, Das UG, Hay WW Jr, Devaskar SU. Glucose transporter protein responses to selective hyperglycemia or hyperinsulinemia in fetal sheep. Am J Phys. 2001;281:R1545–52.
28. Hay WW Jr, Sparks JW, Wilkening RB, Battaglia FC, Meschia G. Fetal glucose uptake and utilization as functions of maternal glucose concentration. Am J Phys. 1984;246:E237–42.
29. Kalhan SC, Savin SM, Adam PAJ. Measurement of glucose turnover in the human newborn with glucose-1–13C. J Clin Endocrinol Metab. 1976;43:704–7.

30. Zarlengo KM, Battaglia FC, Fennessey P, Hay WW Jr. Relationship between glucose utilization rate and glucose concentration in preterm infants. Biol Neonate. 1986;49:181–9.
31. Hay WW Jr, Brown LD, Thorn S, Rozance PJ. Nutrition and development of the fetus: carbohydrate and lipid metabolism (Chapter 27). In: Duggan CP, Watkins JB, Koletzko B, Walker WA, editors. Nutrition in pediatrics (basic science and clinical applications). 5th ed. Shelton: People's Medical Publishing House-USA; 2016. p. 445–63.
32. Aldoretta PW, Carver TD, Hay WW Jr. Maturation of glucose-stimulated insulin secretion. Biol Neonate. 1998;73:375–86. Nicolini U, Hubinont C, Santolaya J, Fisk NM, Rodeck CH. Effects of fetal intravenous glucose challenge in normal and growth retarded fetuses. Horm Metab Res 1990;22:426–430.
33. Carver TD, Anderson SM, Aldoretta PW, Esler AL, Hay WW Jr. Glucose suppression of insulin secretion in chronically hyperglycemic fetal sheep. Pediatr Res. 1995;38:754–62.
34. Carver TD, Anderson SM, Aldoretta PW, Hay WW Jr. Effect of low-level plus marked 'pulsatile' hyperglycemia on insulin secretion in fetal sheep. Am J Phys. 1996;271:E865–71.
35. Frost MS, Zehri AH, Limesand SW, et al. Differential effects of chronic pulsatile versus chronic constant maternal hyperglycemia on fetal pancreatic β-cells. J Pregnancy. 2012;2012:812094.
36. Freinkel N, Phelps NL, Metzger BE. Intermediary metabolism during normal pregnancy. In: Sutherland HW, Stowers JM, editors. Carbohydrate metabolism in pregnancy and the newborn. New York: Springer-Verlag; 1979. p. 1–31.
37. Lavezzi JR, Thorn SR, O'Meara MC, LoTurco D, Brown LD, Hay WW Jr, Rozance PJ. Increased fetal insulin concentrations for one week fail to improve insulin secretion or β-cell mass in fetal sheep with chronically reduced glucose supply. Am J Physiol Regul Integr Comp Physiol. 2013;304:R50–8.
38. Davis MA, Camacho LE, Anderson MJ, Steffens NR, Pendleton AL, Kelly AC, Limesand SW. Chronically elevated norepinephrine concentrations lower glucose uptake in fetal sheep. Am J Physiol Regul Integr Comp Physiol. 2020;319:R255–63.
39. Limesand SW, Rozance PJ. Fetal adaptations in insulin secretion result from high catecholamines during placental insufficiency. J Physiol. 2017;595:5103–13.
40. Limesand SW, Rozance PJ, Smith D, Hay WW Jr. Increased insulin sensitivity and maintenance of glucose utilization rates in fetal sheep with placental insufficiency and intrauterine growth restriction. Am J Physiol Endocrinol Metab. 2007;293:E1716–25.
41. Thorn SR, Rozance PJ, Brown LD, Hay WW Jr. The intrauterine growth restriction phenotype: fetal adaptations and potential implications for later life insulin resistance and diabetes. Semin Reprod Med. 2011;29:225–36.
42. Brown LD, Hay WW Jr. Effect of hyperinsulinemia on amino acid und oxidation independent of glucose metabolism in the ovine fetus. Am J Physiol Endocrinol Metab. 2006;291:E1333–40.
43. Thorn SR, Brown LD, Rozance PJ, Hay WW Jr, Friedman JE. Increased hepatic glucose production in fetal sheep with intrauterine growth restriction is not suppressed by insulin. Diabetes. 2013;62:65–73.
44. Jones AK, Rozance PJ, Brown LD, Goldstrohm DA, Hay WW Jr, Limesand SW, Wesolowski SR. Sustained hypoxemia in late gestation potentiates hepatic gluconeogenic gene expression but does not activate glucose production in the ovine fetus. Am J Physiol Endocrinol Metab. 2019;317:E1–E10.
45. Limesand SW. Gestational diabetes-induced programming of pancreatic islets. Endocrinology. 2019;160:2117–8.
46. DiGiacomo JE, Hay WW Jr. Fetal glucose metabolism and oxygen consumption during sustained maternal and fetal hypoglycemia. Metabolism. 1990;39:193–202.
47. Limesand SW, Rozance PJ, Brown LD, Hay WW Jr. Effects of chronic hypoglycemia and euglycemic correction on lysine metabolism in fetal sheep. Am J Physiol Endocrinol Metab. 2009;296:E879–87.
48. Marconi A, Cetin E, Davoli A, Baggiani AM, Fanelli R, Fennessey PV, Battaglia FC, Pardi G. An evaluation of fetal glucogenesis in intrauterine growth retarded pregnancies: steady

state fetal and maternal enrichments of plasma glucose at cordocentesis. Metabolism. 1993;42:860–4.
49. Hay WW Jr, Sparks JW, Quissell BJ, Battaglia FC, Meschia G. Simultaneous measurements of umbilical glucose uptake, fetal utilization rate, and fetal turnover rate of glucose. Am J Phys. 1981;240:E662–8.
50. Gleason CA, Rudolph AM. Gluconeogenesis by the fetal sheep liver in vivo. J Dev Physiol. 1985;7:185–94.
51. Rozance PJ, Limesand SW, Barry JS, Brown LD, Thorn SR, LoTurco D, Regnault TR, Friedman JE, Hay WW Jr. Chronic late-gestation hypoglycemia upregulates hepatic PEPCK associated with increased PGC1alpha mRNA and phosphorylated CREB in fetal sheep. Am J Physiol Endocrinol Metab. 2008;294:E365–70.
52. Fowden AL, Hill DJ. Intrauterine programming of the endocrine pancreas. Br Med Bull. 2001;60:123–42.
53. Hay WW Jr. Placental function. In: Gluckman PD, Heymann MA, editors. Pediatrics and perinatology: the scientific basis. 2nd ed. London: Edward Arnold; 1996. p. 213–27.

Chapter 3
Normal Neonatal Glucose Metabolism

David H. Adamkin and William W. Hay, Jr.

The management of blood or plasma glucose concentration in the first 48 h of life is one of the most frequently encountered challenges that the healthcare provider faces in the newborn nursery [1–3]. Unfortunately, the plasma concentrations of glucose upon which clinicians base their decision making for treating low glucose concentrations remain more of a matter of expert opinion rather than being evidence-based. Figure 3.1 shows what many would consider a reasonably normal set of data for blood glucose concentrations in normal term neonates over the first 7 days after birth.

The data needed to establish a consensus opinion on blood glucose concentrations that should be treated in the newborn, however, are still not definitive [4]. A review of glucose metabolism right after birth provides an understanding of how complex it is to clearly establish and maintain normal glucose concentrations, particularly above the critical glucose thresholds below which injury may occur [5].

Postnatal Glucose Metabolism

At birth the infant is removed abruptly from its glucose supply and blood glucose concentration decreases. This phenomenon is ubiquitous among mammals and is a normal physiological function that is essential for activating glucose production by the neonate. Several hormonal and metabolic changes at birth facilitate adaptations that provide glucose to replace the supply previously received via the placenta. Induction of HGP begins shortly before term birth and is augmented after birth by

D. H. Adamkin (✉)
Division of Neonatal Medicine, University of Louisville, Louisville, Kentucky, USA
e-mail: david.adamkin@louisville.edu

W. W. Hay, Jr.
University of Colorado, Denver, CO, USA

D. H. Adamkin, W. W. Hay, Jr. (eds.), *Disorders of Neonatal Glycemia*,
https://doi.org/10.1007/978-3-032-29094-6_3

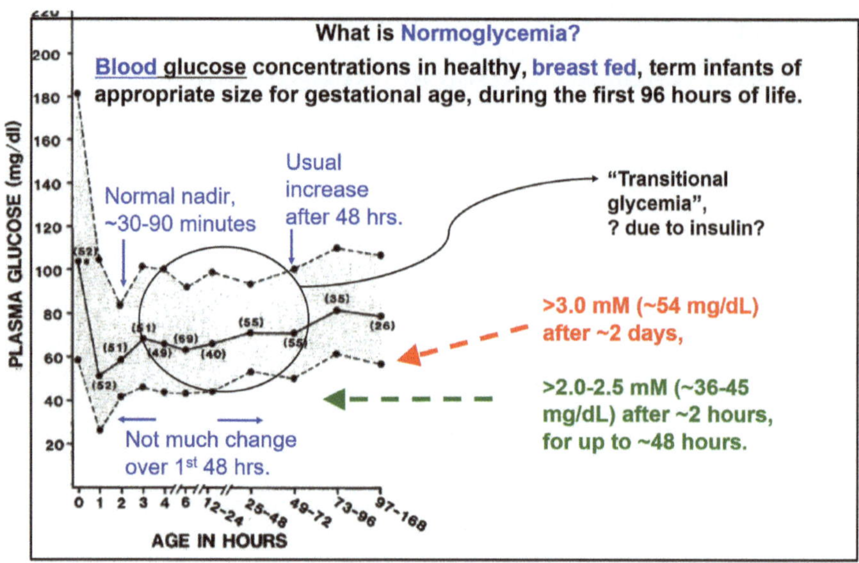

Fig. 3.1 What is Normoglycemia? 95% of normal term AGA neonates have a plasma glucose values are greater than 40–45 mg/dL (>2.2–2.5 mmol/L) after the first 2–3 h of life through 24–48 h, increasing to greater than 54 mg/dL (3.0 mmol/L) after 24–48 h. (Adapted from Refs. [1–3])

increased secretion of glucagon and glucocorticoids that trigger gene transcription of PEPCK and activate gluconeogenesis [6, 7]. Catecholamine concentrations increase markedly at birth and together with glucagon activate hepatic glycogen phosphorylase and glycogenolysis. The perinatal surge in fetal cortisol secretion stimulates hepatic glucose-6-phosphatase activity and hepatic glucose release. Increased catecholamines also stimulate lipolysis, providing energy (ATP) and cofactors (NADPH) that enhance activity of enzymes responsible for gluconeogenesis.

Blood or plasma glucose concentrations fall after birth from the normal fetal concentrations, reaching a nadir around 30 min to 1½ h of age, followed by a gradual increase after 24–48 h to normal values found in healthy, non-stressed, term, breast fed infants. Normal glucose concentrations range from about 54 mg/dL (~3 mmol/L) to about 108 mg/dL (6 mmol/L). These normal values are achieved by a balance of neonatal hepatic glucose production rates and glucose utilization rates throughout the body, although most glucose consumption occurs in the brain (Table 3.1).

Maintenance of Glucose Homeostasis

Maintenance of glucose homeostasis depends on the balance between hepatic glucose output and peripheral glucose utilization. Steady state glucose utilization rates in term neonates are 3–5 mg/min/kg, about half the values of 8–9 mg/min/kg that

Table 3.1 Endocrine, metabolic, biochemical, and physiological changes that occur at the time of birth that allow a normal term newborn to produce and maintain normal circulating glucose concentrations

1. Insulin declines, leading to increased glucose production via glycogenolysis (early) and gluconeogenesis (later) and decreased peripheral glucose utilization in insulin sensitive tissues (largely skeletal muscle and heart).
2. Glucagon, adrenalin, cortisol, growth hormone, and thyroid stimulating hormone increase, leading to glycogenolysis (via activation of adenylate cyclase), gluconeogenesis (fueled by glycerol, lactate, and amino acids), lipolysis, and lipid oxidation.
3. These hormonal changes lead to increased hepatic glucose release into the circulation and the production of glycerol that fuels gluconeogenesis and free fatty acids and ketones that substitute for glucose in mitochondrial oxidation and energy production.
4. In the absence of pathological conditions and the normal addition of milk via intermittent suckling, the balance of these hormonal and biochemical actions results in normoglycemia (3.0–6.0 mmol/L [54–108 mg/dL]).

Adapted from Ref. [5]

occur at earlier gestational ages in both the fetus and preterm infant of the same gestational age. Peripheral glucose utilization may increase during hypoxia due to the inherent inefficiency of anaerobic glycolysis, hyperinsulinemia which increases glucose uptake by insulin-sensitive tissues, and cold stress which increases metabolic rate via sympathetic nervous system activity and thyroid hormone secretion. Once normal feedings are established, glycerol and amino acids continue to fuel gluconeogenesis. Once milk feedings start, galactose derived from hydrolysis of milk sugar (lactose) in the gut increases hepatic glycogen production and allows for sustained between-feeding hepatic glucose release from glycogen breakdown. Feedings also induce production of intestinal peptides, or incretins, that promote insulin secretion. Insulin decreases hepatic glucose production and increases glucose utilization for energy production and storage as glycogen. If rates of glycogenolysis and gluconeogenesis do not match the rate of glucose utilization because of failure of hormonal control mechanisms or reduced alternate substrate supply, disturbances of glucose homeostasis develop, including hypoglycemia.

Glucose Production and Utilization Rates in Normal Neonates

After birth, blood glucose production is primarily a function of the liver. The complexities of postnatal glucose metabolic adaptation include the induction of hepatic glycogenolysis and gluconeogenesis and interplay of insulin, glucagon, catecholamines, corticosteroids, and other hormones [8–12]. Brain glucose utilization is the major determinant of (hepatic) glucose production [13]. Glucose production rates among infants and children from 1 to 25 kg body weight are twofold to threefold greater than older subjects on a body weight basis. Such rates have been measured using tracer methodology with an infusion of nonradioactive stable isotopes of glucose [13, 14]. These higher rates occur because the neonatal brain to body weight ratio is much higher than in adults (Fig. 3.2).

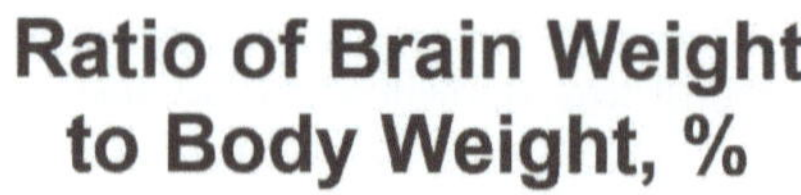

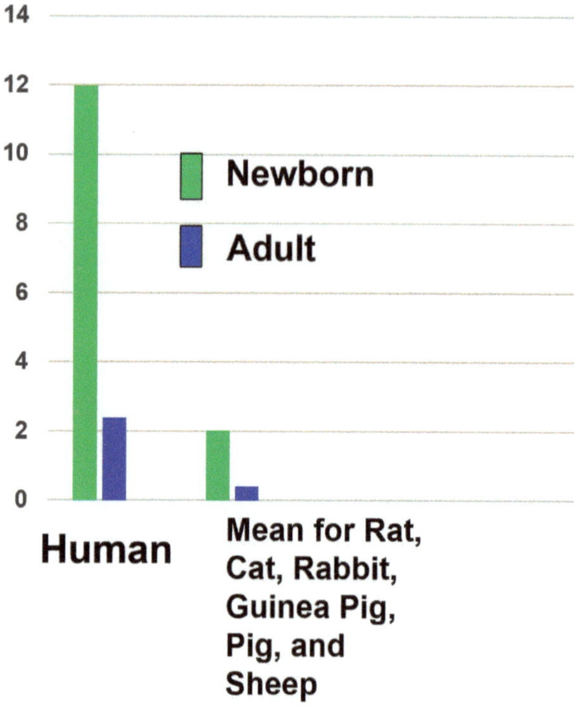

Fig. 3.2 Human newborns are unique among mammals in having a much higher brain/body weight ratio, and the brain requires glucose for its normal function. (Adapted from: Cross [15] and as noted in Ref. [15], adapted from original data in Altman and Dittmer [16] and as adapted from Potter [17])

Body weight-specific glucose utilization rates can be higher in preterm infants and IUGR infants who have a greater brain to body weight ratio than normal term infants, often as high as 5–7 mg/min/kg. Likewise, body weight-specific glucose utilization rates can be lower in obese, macrosomic infants, such as infants of diabetic mothers (IDMs), who have a lower brain to body weight ratio and a large fat mass that has low rates of glucose uptake and metabolism.

The relationship between glucose utilization and brain size is linear, demonstrating that the disproportionately greater rates of glucose production and utilization in the neonatal period relate to the larger neonatal brain. Additionally, central nervous system consumption of glucose accounts for the majority of total hepatic glucose output in the preterm infants. However, maximal glucose uptake in these infants is approximately one third to one half of the comparable values for mature brain, indicating a reduced number of available luminal transporters [14]. Because brain glucose uptake is concentration gradient (plasma to brain extracellular fluid) determined, plasma glucose concentration is a critical regulator of brain glucose concentration and brain glucose uptake. For example, extrapolation of the reversible Michaelis-Menten model to hypoglycemia predicts the plasma glucose concentration (2.1 ± 0.6 mmol/L) at which brain glucose concentrations approach zero. At this point, cerebral blood flow increases sharply by 57% ± 22%, indicating that brain glucose concentration, and thus plasma glucose concentration, is the signal that triggers defense mechanisms aimed at ensuring glucose delivery to the brain during hypoglycemia [18].

Glucose is the primary fuel to produce chemical energy that is essential for maintenance of normal brain function [19–21]. The respiratory quotient of the brain is approximately 1. This indicates that carbohydrate, principally glucose, as well as its metabolic product, lactate, is the major substrate oxidized by neural tissue. Glucose is the only carbohydrate extracted by the brain in any significant amount. Also, cerebral glucose uptake is almost completely accounted for by cerebral oxygen uptake. As a result, central nervous system function is rapidly and negatively impacted by hypoglycemia.

Alternative Glucose Substrates

Alternative substrates for glucose in brain metabolism can be used for energy production and other metabolic processes. Under normal circumstances, such alternatives are probably not of major importance for energy production. However, in conditions in which glucose is limited (e.g. hypoglycemia), alternative substrates may support brain oxidative metabolism, function, and structure. These alternative substrates include lactate, pyruvate, free fatty acids, glycerol, a variety of ketoacids (i.e. ketone bodies), and certain amino acids. These alternative substrates are capable of partially or completely supporting respiration of brain tissue slices in in vitro studies. Certain of these substrates are produced in the brain during hypoglycemia. These include amino acids from the degradation of protein and fatty acids from the degradation of phospholipid. They are potentially used as alternative energy sources. These latter alternative sources are, however, not optimal because their sources are largely structural (protein and phospholipids) components. Conservation of energy production at the price of brain structure is not a desirable or successful adaptive response. Also, the systemically derived alternative substrates either do not appear in appreciable quantities in blood or cannot cross the blood brain barrier to a significant extent. Thus, they cannot contribute much to brain energy requirements when hypoglycemia occurs. Lactate and ketone bodies are the two substrates for which data shows value for the support of oxidative metabolism in the neonatal brain when hypoglycemia occurs [19, 20, 21–24].

Healthy term infants with hypoglycemia have a variable number of alternative fuels. Specifically, lactate contributes approximately 25% of the potential adenosine triphosphate (ATP) in the first 24 h and is the largest source of energy other than glucose, which provides 72–84% of ATP production. Unfortunately, ketone production now has been shown to only contribute to ATP beginning on days 2–3 and only provides 7% of potential ATP production. Ketone body production is even further limited and is inversely related to gestational age [25]. Physiological transition is associated with increased cerebral blood flow as glucose concentrations decrease.

This increases the delivery of essential energy sources for the brain with glucose and lactate, and with more maturity after birth and enteral feeding also included ketones [26–30].

References

1. Perlman JM, Volpe JJ. Glucose, Chapter 25. In: Volpe JJ, Inder TE, Darras BT, de Vries LS, du Plessis AJ, Neil J, Perlman JM, editors. Neurology of the newborn. 6th ed. Elsevier; 2018. p. 701–29.
2. Srinivasan G, Pildes RS, Cattamanchi G, Voora S, Lilien LD. Plasma glucose values in normal neonates: a new look. J Pediatr. 1986;109:114–7.
3. Hoseth E, Joergensen A, Ebbesen F, Moeller M. Blood glucose levels in a population of healthy, breast fed, term infants of appropriate size for gestational age. Arch Dis Child Fetal Neonatal Ed. 2000;83:F117–9.
4. Adamkin DH. Neonatal hypoglycemia. In: Martin GI, Rosenfeld W, editors. Common problems in the newborn nursery, an evidence and care based guide. Cham: Springer; 2019. p. 99–108.
5. Guemes M, Rahman W, Hussain K. What is a normal blood glucose? Arch Dis Child. 2016;101:569–74.
6. Girard J. Metabolic adaptations to change of nutrition at birth. Biol Neonate. 1990;58(Suppl 1):3–15.
7. Fowden AL, Mundy L, Silver M. Developmental regulation of glucogenesis in the sheep fetus during late gestation. J Physiol. 1998;508:937–47.
8. Hawdon JM, Aynsley-Green A, Alberti KG, Ward Platt MP. The role of pancreatic insulin secretion in neonatal glucoregulation. I. Healthy term and preterm infants. Arch Dis Child. 1993;68:274–3.
9. Hawdon JM, Ward Platt MP. Metabolic adaptation in small for gestational age infants. Arch Dis Child. 1993;68:262–79.
10. Hawdon JM, Weddell, Aynsley-Green, Ward Platt MP. Hormonal and metabolic response to hypoglycemia in small for gestational age infants. Arch Dis Child. 1993;68:269–73.
11. Hawdon JM, Aynsley-Green A, Ward Platt MP. Neonatal blood concentrations: metabolic effects of intravenous glucagon and intragastric medium chain triglyceride. Arch Dis Child. 1993;68:255–61.
12. Hawdon JM, Aynsley-Green A, Bartlett K, Ward Platt MP. The role of pancreatic insulin secretion in neonatal glucoregulation. II. Infants with disordered blood glucose homeostasis. Arch Dis Child. 1993;68:280–5.
13. Bier DM, Leake RD, Haymond MW, Arnold KJ, Gruenke LD, Sperling MA, Kipnis DM. Measurement of "true" glucose production rates in infancy and childhood with 6-6 dideuteroglucose. Diabetes. 1977;26:1016–23.
14. Powers WJ, Rosenbaum JL, Dence CS, Markham J, Videen TO. Cerebral glucose transport and metabolism in preterm infants. J Cereb Blood Flow Metab. 1998;18:632–8.
15. Cross KW. Review Lecture. La Chaleur Animale and the infant brain. J Physiol. 1979;294:1–21.
16. Altman PL, Dittmer DS. Growth including reproduction and morphological development. In: Zweimer RL, editor. Fed Am Socs Exp Biol, biological handbook. Washington, DC: Nat Acad Sci; 1962. p. 358.
17. Potter EL. Pathology of the foetus and the newborn. Chicago: Yearbook Publishers Inc.; 1953.
18. Choi IY, Lee SP, Kim SG, Gruetter R. In vivo measurements of brain glucose transport using the reversible Michaelis-Menten model and simultaneous measurements of cerebral blood flow changes during hypoglycemia. J Cereb Blood Flow Metab. 2001;21:653–63.

19. Vanuci RC. Cerebral carbohydrate and energy metabolism in perinatal hypoxic ischemic brain damage. Brain Pathol. 1992;2:229–34.
20. Nehlig A, Periera de Vasconcelos A. Glucose and ketone body utilization by the brain of neonatal rats. Prog Neurobiol. 1993;40:163–221.
21. Hernandez MJ, Vanucci RC, Salcedo A, Brennan RW. Cerebral blood flow and metabolism during hypoglycemia in newborn dogs. J Neurochem. 1989;35:622–8.
22. Dombrowski GJ, Swiatek KR, Chao KL. Lactate, 3-hydroxybutyrate, and glucose as substrates for the early postnatal rat brain. Neurochem Res. 1989;14:667–75.
23. Young RS, Petroff OA, Chen B, Aquila WJ Jr, Gore JC. Preferential utilization of lactate in neonatal dog brain: in vivo and in vitro proton NMR study. Biol Neonate. 1991;59:46–53.
24. Thurston JH, Hauhart RE, Schro J. Beta hydroxybutyrate reverses insulin induced hypoglycemia coma in suckling weaning mice despite low blood and brain glucose levels. Metab Brain Dis. 1968;1:63–81.
25. Harris DL, Weston PJ, Harding JE. Lactate rather than ketones may provide alternative fuel in hypoglycemic newborns. Arch Dis Child Fetal Neonatal Ed. 2015;100:F161–4.
26. De Boisseue D, Rocchiccioli F, Kalach N, Bougneres PF. Ketone body turnover at term and in premature newborns in the first two weeks after birth. Biol Neonate. 1995;67:84–93.
27. Pryds O, Christensen NJ, Friss-Hansen B. Increased cerebral blood flow and plasma epinephrine in hypoglycemic preterm infants. Pediatrics. 1990;85:172–6.
28. Matterberger C, Baik-Schneditz N, Schwarberger B, Schmölzer GM, Mileder L, Pichler-Stachl E, Urlesberger B, Pichler G. Blood glucose and cerebral oxygenation immediately after birth: an observations study. J Pediatrics. 2018;200:19–23.
29. Anwar M, Vanucci RC. Autoradiographic determination of regional cerebral blood flow during hypoglycemia in newborn dogs. J Ped Res. 1988;24:41–5.
30. Vanderhaegen J, Vanhaesebrouck S, Vanhole C, Caesar P, Naulers G. The effect of glycemia on the cerebral oxygenation in very low birthweight infants as measured by near infra-red spectroscopy. Adv Exp Med Biol. 2010;662:461–6.

Part III
Neonatal Hypoglycemia

Chapter 4
Conditions in the Fetus that Promote Neonatal Hypoglycemia

William W. Hay, Jr.

Increased Insulin Production in Fetuses of Diabetic Mothers and Propensity for Neonatal Hypoglycemia

Classic studies over 70 years ago by Jørgen Pederson determined that higher maternal glucose concentrations in pregnant women with insulin-dependent diabetes produce hyperglycemia in the fetus, inducing increased insulin secretion in the fetus and the development of macrosomia, primarily due to increased fat production in adipose tissue. In these fetuses, pancreatic islet hyperplasia developed that persisted after birth, leading to often profound and persistent neonatal hypoglycemia when maternal and placental glucose supplies stopped at birth and often feedings of the infant were delayed [1–3]. Because most of these infants were otherwise healthy at birth, their catecholamine concentrations decreased after birth, reducing catecholamine suppression of insulin secretion [4–6]. The same problem is now highly exaggerated globally with the development of obesity in pregnancy and gestational diabetes. Both of these conditions involve maternal and thus fetal hyperglycemia, fetal hyperinsulinemia, neonatal hyperinsulinemia, and neonatal hypoglycemia [7].

While constant, high glucose concentrations in the pregnant diabetic mother and thus the fetus over long periods may decrease GSIS, [8] as shown in in vivo experiments in maternal and fetal sheep, acute spikes or pulses of high glucose concentrations (pulsatile hyperglycemia) increase fetal insulin secretion [9, 10]. In humans, this can occur with high sugar meals and snacks, in addition to meals that are rich in glucose and easily digestible carbohydrates, which is common in GDMs in whom there is a strong tendency to develop increasingly exaggerated, meal-associated, "pulsatile" hyperglycemia in late gestation and associated increases in fetal and neonatal insulin secretion (Fig. 4.1) [11–14].

W. W. Hay, Jr. (✉)
University of Colorado, Denver, CO, USA
e-mail: bill.hay@ucdenver.edu

D. H. Adamkin, W. W. Hay, Jr. (eds.), *Disorders of Neonatal Glycemia*,
https://doi.org/10.1007/978-3-032-29094-6_4

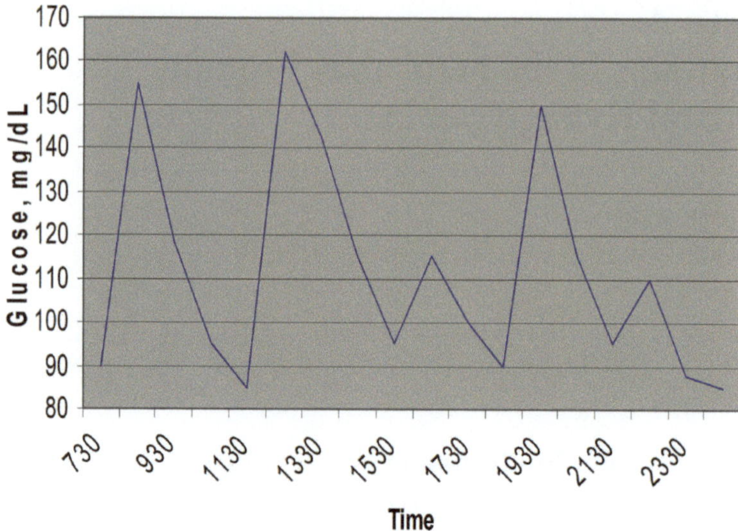

Fig. 4.1 24 hour maternal glucose concentration variations in response to intermittent food intake and fasting. (Figure drawn by Dr. Teri Hernandez, University of Colorado School of Nursing, adapted from data in: Hernandez et al. [12]; Barbour et al. [13])

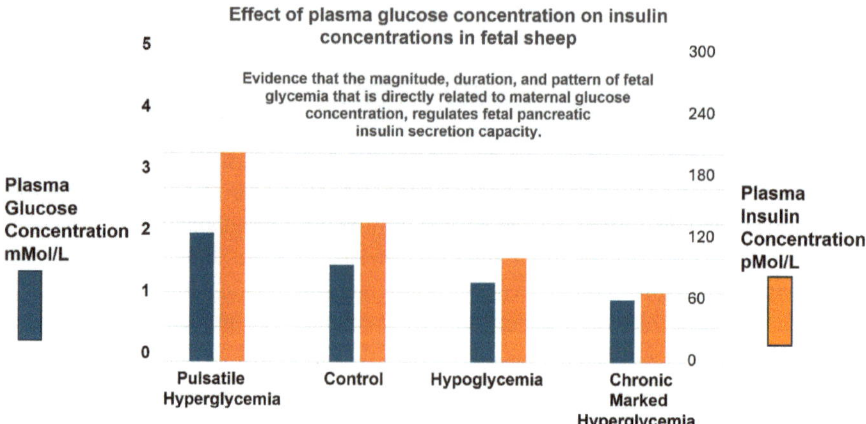

Fig. 4.2 Pulsatile hyperglycemia induces the greatest increase in insulin secretion in contrast to constant, marked hyperglycemia that suppresses insulin secretion. (Adapted from Carver et al. [9])

When studied in a controlled animal model, the pregnant sheep, fetal glucose-stimulated insulin secretion (GSIS) is most augmented by pulsatile hyperglycemia that is characteristic of gestational diabetics and milder but poorly controlled insulin dependent diabetics [8–10]. Hypoglycemia suppresses GSIS, but chronic, marked hyperglycemia has the greatest suppression of GSIS. Thus, the magnitude, duration, and pattern of fetal glycemia, directly regulated by maternal plasma glucose concentration, regulates fetal pancreatic insulin secretion capacity [11] (Fig. 4.2, [9]).

At birth, glucose supply to the neonate stops when the umbilical cord is cut, separating the infant from the constant supply of glucose via the placenta from the maternal circulation. IDMs have abundant, often exaggerated fat and glycogen stores that normally could support oxidative metabolism in addition to glucose, but these infants often are less capable than normal infants of mobilizing these substrate stores. Insulin secretion is thus in excess and quickly decreases glucose production and increases glucose utilization, as well as amino acid and fatty acids, in insulin sensitive tissues (primarily skeletal muscle, heart, and adipose tissue) [15, 16].

Normal neonates quickly mobilize hepatic glycogen after birth in response to catecholamines and falling glucose concentrations to maintain plasma glucose concentration [17]. This increases insulin secretion, however, which in turn inhibits glycogenolysis by specifically blocking glycogen phosphorylase enzyme activity. Insulin also inhibits the normal postnatal activation of phosphoenolpyruvate carboxykinase (PEPCK), the rate-limiting enzyme of gluconeogenesis, by glucagon and cortisol as plasma glucose concentrations decrease. Fatty acids released from fat cells by catecholamines are oxidized, as are ketones (though they are usually low until after feeding). Both are important for the maintenance of normal glucose concentrations.

Frequently, these processes are impaired in IDMs by their high fetal and thus early neonatal insulin concentrations. Insulin also promotes the production of malonyl Co-A and acetyl Co-A carboxylase activity, which promotes glucose oxidation, inhibits fatty acid oxidation, and re-directs fatty acids into synthetic pathways. Hyperinsulinism in fetal IDMs also inhibits free fatty acid release from fat cells in competition with their release by catecholamines and limits the availability of fatty acids as an alternative substrates for oxidative metabolism. Glucose is then used more quickly, contributing to tendencies for hypoglycemia. Ketone production from fatty acids is decreased for the same reasons, decreasing their availability for energy production. These processes lead to increased glucose utilization, decreased glucose production, and decreased availability of alternate oxidative substrates. Some recent studies, however, have shown that despite increased insulin concentrations, lipolysis (as measured by glycerol production) in a small group of IDMs was unimpaired and the gluconeogenic contribution from glycerol was higher than in healthy newborns [18–20]. One should not assume, however, that IDMs can mount adequate alternative energy substrate production (FFAs, ketoacids) during episodes of low glucose concentrations.

Persistent Hyperinsulinism-Like Hypoglycemia in IUGR Infants

Why do preterm and particularly IUGR neonates become hypoglycemic, often persistently and despite early IV dextrose and early enteral feeding? This condition, generally called "transitional hypoglycemia" is relatively common and has only recently garnered sufficient and new basic and clinical research to resolve how it develops, how it contributes to low glucose concentrations in primarily IUGR infants, and how it should be screened for and treated [21–24].

Formerly, and commonly (as written in textbooks), this condition was believed to be related to limited glycogen and fat stores especially in the initial days of extra-uterine life [25]. Many also assumed that these infants experience impaired glycogenolysis, secondary to low glycogen stores and impaired gluconeogenesis, secondary to delayed induction of enzymes [26]. But as discussed in Part IV, glucose production develops immediately after birth even in very preterm infants, and as shown in Fig. 4.3, glucose production is supported by normal amounts of hepatic glycogen and the principal enzyme, phosphoenolpyruvate carboxy kinas (PEPCK) that activates gluconeogenesis [27–33]. Clearly, even IUGR fetuses can have relatively normal amounts of hepatic glucogenic capacity. The notion that they cannot produce glucose into their circulation in sufficient amounts to support vital oxidative metabolism is not necessary the case.

Transitional hypoglycemia is a common, self-limiting condition in newborns (0–48 h) caused by a temporary, physiologically lower threshold for insulin suppression, often resulting in blood glucose levels below 40–50 mg/dL. The Pediatric Endocrine Society (PES) emphasizes differentiating this from persistent, pathological hypoglycemia (e.g., genetic hyperinsulinism) by assessing for symptomatic, prolonged, or recurrent low glucose levels that require intravenous treatment, typically resolving within 72–96 h [34]. This condition has several components as well as a relatively increased insulin/glucose concentration ratio:

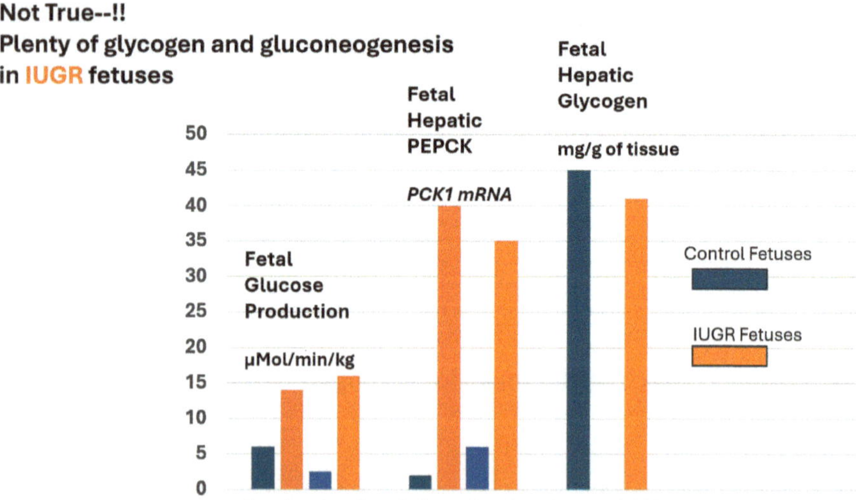

Fig. 4.3 Fetal glucose production and hepatic PEPCK and glycogen content in chronically IUGR fetal sheep [32, 33]

1. Greater head/brain to body/liver ratio, thus greater body weight-specific glucose utilization rates (Fig. 4.4). Obviously, this condition persists well after birth.
2. Fetal Glucose Utilization Rates in sheep at ~75 days or ~50% of gestation is normally quite high, around 9.4 mg/kg/min. By 140 days or about 93% of gestation, GUR is lower at about 4.9 mg/kg/min, relatively lower by the growth of internal organs that don't use as much glucose as the brain, such as bone, fat, and muscle. IUGR fetuses, even close to term, are more like fetuses at mid-gestation, as they develop without as much bone or fat or muscle as normal fetuses do [35].
3. Increased peripheral tissue glucose uptake capacity, from increased or at least maintained glucose transporters (Fig. 4.5). These conditions maintain glucose utilization and insulin sensitivity, i.e., GUR/kg body weight is normal, about the same as normally grown fetuses of the same gestational age, but at less than normal fetal plasma glucose and insulin concentrations [36]. This condition persists well after birth.
4. The IUGR fetus has lower glucose and oxygen supplies, plasma glucose concentrations, and blood oxygen content. These conditions stimulate catecholamine production that attenuates basal and glucose-stimulated insulin secretion (Fig. 4.6).
5. The IUGR fetus appears to adapt to the lower glucose concentrations and has a lower set point for glucose concentration [37]. The mean plasma glucose concentration in these infants below which insulin secretion decreases is 55–65 mg/

IUGR fetuses have a greater head/brain to body/liver ratio, thus greater body weight-specific glucose utilization rates.

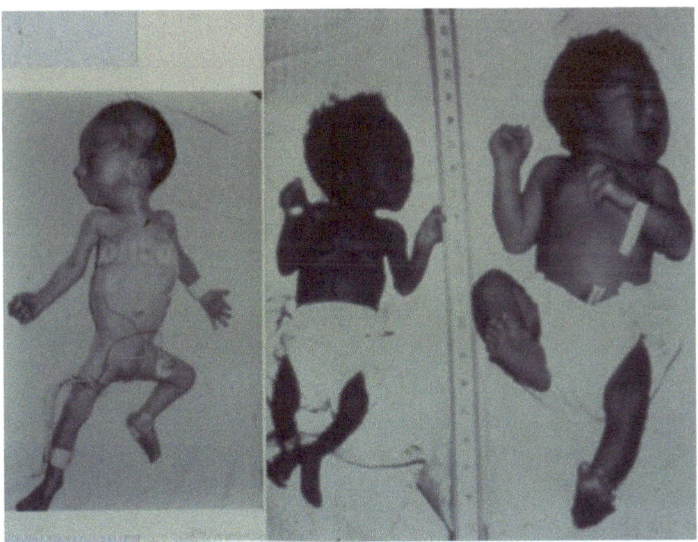

Fig. 4.4 A greater head/brain to body/liver size ratio is obvious in the extremely to very preterm infant on the left and the late preterm IUGR infant in the middle compared with the term AGA infant on the right. (From The National Archives)

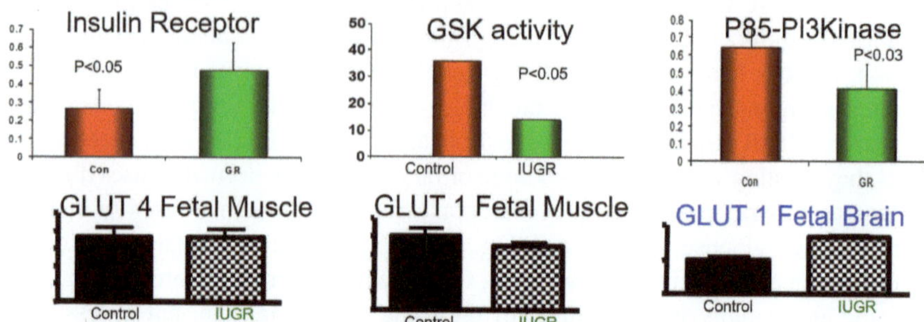

Fig. 4.5 Reduced oxygen and nutrient supply to the IUGR fetus induces up-regulation of glucose utilization and insulin sensitivity [36]

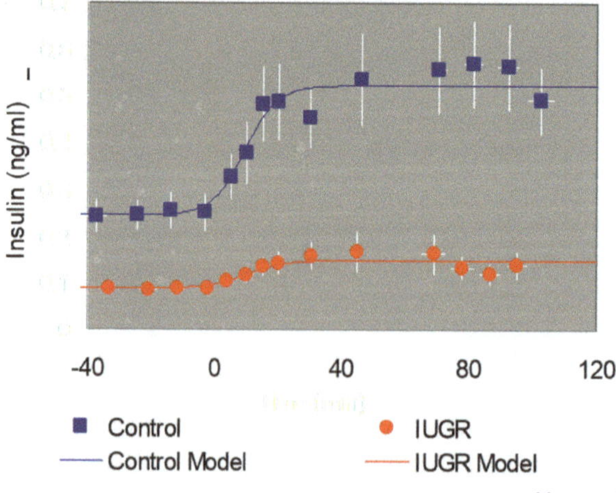

Fig. 4.6 Glucose stimulated insulin secretion is reduced in IUGR fetal sheep that are relatively hypoxic [4]

dL (3.1–3.6 mM) in the first 48 h of life, and lower glucose concentrations do not appear to decrease insulin concentrations as much as in older infants or children (i.e., this is a higher insulin/glucose ratio than normal—"relative hyperinsulinemia"). "Hyperinsulinemia" in newborns is transient and normally "resolves" by 2–4 days of age. This condition develops at least in part, as fetal hypoxia and reduced nutrient supply from reduced placental oxygen and nutrient transport increases fetal catecholamine secretion that suppresses fetal pancreatic β-cell insulin production and secretion.

6. At the same time, there is an increase in the fraction of insulin that is secreted in response to glucose and other insulin secretagogues (Fig. 4.7). This condition persists well after birth [36–38].
7. After birth, with normalization of neonatal blood oxygen supply and PaO_2, there is increased insulin secretion after reduction of catecholamines and their suppression of insulin secretion. This has been tested in the IUGR fetal sheep by infusing blockers of catecholamines that then results in increased insulin secretion (Fig. 4.8) [2, 39], and by infusing norepinephrine into normal fetuses that suppresses their insulin secretion (Fig. 4.9) [39].

   This happens under basal, low glucose conditions and hyperglycemic conditions, proving that the suppression of fetal insulin secretion is produced by increased catecholamines [6]. After birth, if hypoxia or stress continues to stimulate catecholamine secretion, insulin secretion will remain suppressed, leading to hyperglycemia, particularly when dextrose is infused intravenously [39].

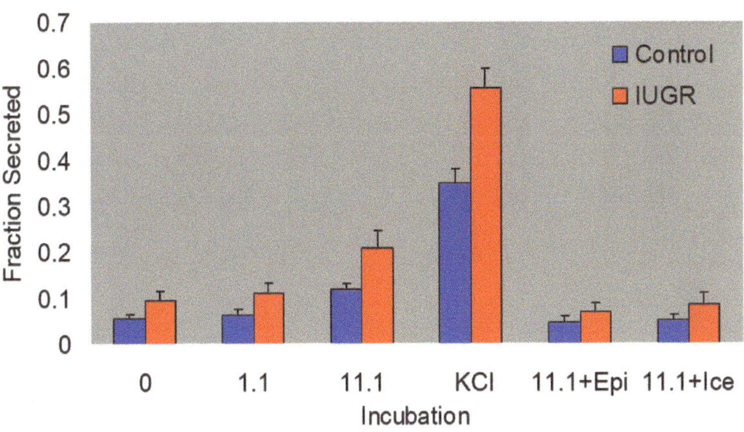

Fig. 4.7 Increased pancreatic islet fractional insulin secretion capacity develops after hypoxia-induced suppression of insulin secretion in IUGR fetal sheep [38]

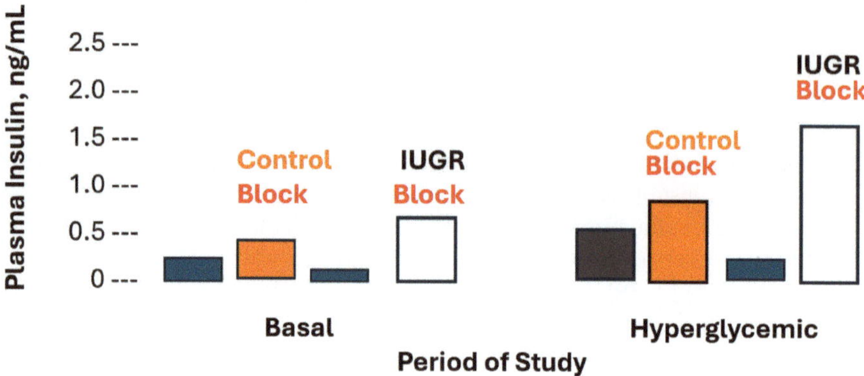

Fig. 4.8 Blocking hypoxia-induced increased catecholamines promotes insulin secretion. (Adapted from: Leos et al. [6])

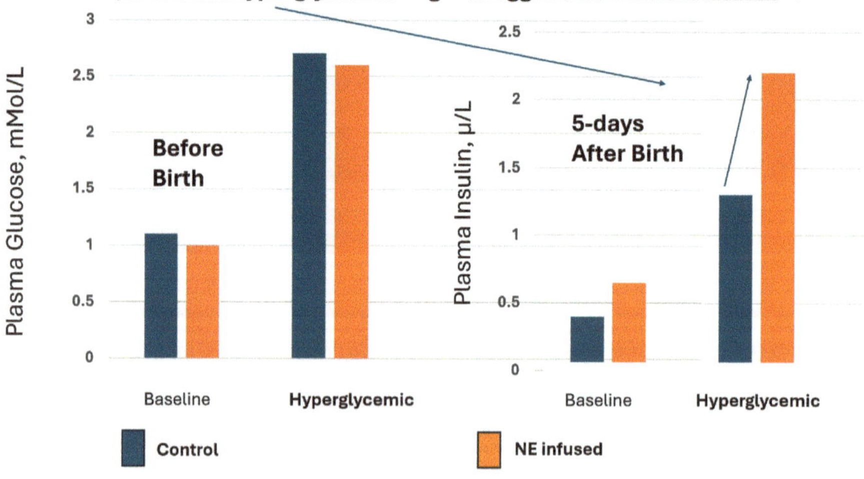

Fig. 4.9 Persistent increase in glucose stimulated insulin secretion following norepinephrine infusion [39]

8. After birth, as soon as catecholamines are reduced, the increased pancreatic insulin secretion adaptation that occurred in the fetus leads to increased fractional insulin secretion that then can result in hypoglycemia, particularly when glucose supply is limited (feedings are delayed and/or IV dextrose infusion is delayed or is too low). This condition persists well after birth, up to 2–4 weeks, when it can lead to increased neonatal glucose utilization rates that further enhance neonatal hypoglycemia (Fig. 4.10) [40].

   While the explanation for this propensity for development of postnatal hypoglycemia in IUGR infants is based on physiological studies in fetal sheep, the persistent hyperinsulin-like hypoglycemia in human IUGR infants is clearly recognized and is a significant clinical problem that can persist well after birth and require careful evaluation and treatment, often with continued IV dextrose infusions and early and frequent feedings [41, 42].

In summary, persistent hyperinsulin-like hypoglycemia in preterm and particularly IUGR infants is a significant clinical problem that results from conditions that developed during fetal life. In such fetuses, their greater head/brain to body/liver ratio produces a greater body weight-specific glucose utilization rate. This needs to be considered when infusing dextrose on a body weight-specific basis. These infants also have increased peripheral tissue glucose uptake capacity from increased glucose transporters or at least glucose transporter number and affinity for glucose despite low plasma glucose and insulin concentrations. Increased susceptibility to anapleurotic metabolic stimulation of fractional insulin secretion uniquely develops in the fetus with suppressed insulin sensitivity from low plasma glucose concentrations and reduced pancreatic islet and β-cell hyperplasia. After birth, sudden increases in plasma glucose concentration can thus promote exaggerated insulin

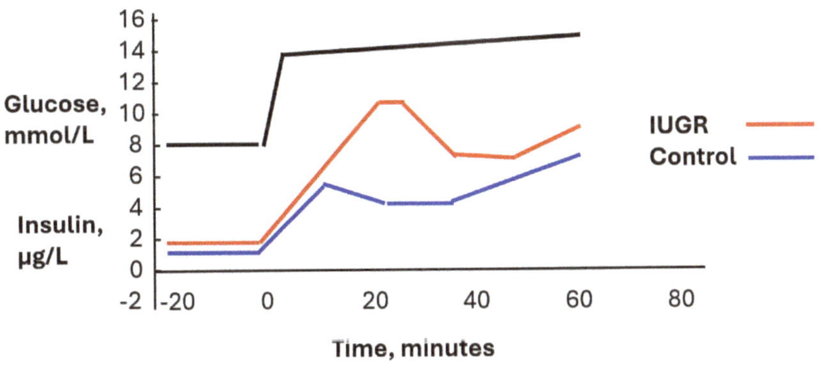

Fig. 4.10 Glucose stimulated insulin secretion persists for up to 1 week after delivery in IUGR lambs [40]

secretion leading to sudden and often profound, as well as persistent hypoglycemia. This is augmented by increased insulin secretion after reduction of catecholamine suppression of insulin secretion, which commonly occurs after birth as the infant is exposed to higher environmental and thus arterial oxygen concentrations. Such infants should be identified early and treated with careful, frequent, and usually small adjustments in IV dextrose infusion rates. Early enteral feeding also is helpful, especially when given in small, frequent amounts.

References

1. Pedersen J. Diabetes and pregnancy: blood sugar of newborn infants. Ph.D. thesis, Danish Science Press, Copenhagen. 1952. p. 230.
2. Pedersen J. The pregnant diabetic and her newborn: problems and management. Baltimore: Williams & Wilkins; 1967. p. 128–37.
3. Schwartz R, Gruppuso PA, Petzold K, Brambilla D, Hiilesmaa V, Teramo KA. Hyperinsulinemia and macrosomia in the fetus of the diabetic mother. Diabetes Care. 1994;17:640–8.
4. Limesand SW, Rozance PJ, Zerbe GO, Hutton JC, Hay WW Jr. Attenuated insulin release and storage in fetal sheep pancreatic islets with intrauterine growth restriction. Endocrinology. 2006;14:1488–97.
5. Andrews SE, Brown LD, Thorn SR, Limesand SW, Davis M, Hay WW Jr, Rozance PJ. Increased adrenergic signaling is responsible for decreased glucose-stimulated insulin secretion in the chronically hyperinsulinemic ovine fetus. Endocrinology. 2015;156:367–76.
6. Leos RA, Anderson MJ, Chen X, Pugmire J, Anderson KA, Limesand SW. Chronic exposure to elevated norepinephrine suppresses insulin secretion in fetal sheep with placental insufficiency and intrauterine growth restriction. Am J Physiol Endocrinol Metab. 2010;298:E770–8.
7. Catalano PM, Hauguel-De Mouzon S. Is it time to revisit the Pedersen hypothesis in the face of the obesity epidemic? Am J Obstet Gynecol. 2011;204:479–87.
8. Carver TD, Anderson SM, Aldoretta PW, Esler AL, Hay WW Jr. Glucose suppression of insulin secretion in chronically hyperglycemic fetal sheep. Pediatr Res. 1995;38:754–62.
9. Carver TD, Anderson SM, Aldoretta PW, Hay WW Jr. Effect of low-level plus marked 'pulsatile' hyperglycemia on insulin secretion in fetal sheep. Am J Phys. 1996;271:E865–71.
10. Frost MS, Zehri AH, Limesand SW, Hay WW Jr, Rozance PJ. Differential effects of chronic pulsatile versus chronic constant maternal hyperglycemia on fetal pancreatic β-cells. J Pregnancy. 2012;2012:812094.
11. Hay WW Jr. Nutrient delivery and metabolism in the fetus. In: Hod M, Jovanovic L, Di Renzo GC, de Leiva A, Langer O, editors. Textbook of diabetes and pregnancy. London: Martin Dunitz; 2003. p. 201.
12. Hernandez TL, Van Pelt RE, Anderson MA, Daniels LJ, West NA, Donahoo WT, Friedman JE, Barbour LA. A higher-complex carbohydrate diet in gestational diabetes mellitus achieves glucose targets and lowers postprandial lipids: a randomized crossover study. Diabetes Care. 2014;37:1254–62.
13. Barbour LA, Farabi SS, Friedman JE, Hirsch NM, Reece MS, Van Pelt RE, Hernandez TL. Postprandial triglycerides predict newborn fat more strongly than glucose in women with obesity in early pregnancy. Obesity (Silver Spring). 2018;26:1347–56.
14. Freinkel N, Phelps NL, Metzger BE. Intermediary metabolism during normal pregnancy. In: Sutherland HW, Stowers JM, editors. Carbohydrate metabolism in pregnancy and the newborn. New York: Springer-Verlag; 1979. p. 1–31.
15. Hay WW Jr. Care of the infant of the diabetic mother. Curr Diab Rep. 2012;12:4–15.

16. Hay WW Jr. Recent observations on the regulation of fetal metabolism by glucose. J Physiol. 2006;572:17–24.
17. Persson B. Neonatal glucose metabolism in offspring of mothers with varying degrees of hyperglycemia during pregnancy. Semin Fetal Neonatal Med. 2009;14:106–10.
18. Gustafsson J. Neonatal energy substrate production. Indian J Med Res. 2009;130:618–23.
19. Sunehag A, Ewald U, Larsson A, Gustafsson J. Attenuated hepatic glucose production but unimpaired lipolysis in newborn infants of mothers with diabetes. Pediatr Res. 1997;42:492–7.
20. Ahlsson FS, Diderholm B, Ewald U, Gustafsson J. Lipolysis and insulin sensitivity at birth in infants who are large for gestational age. Pediatrics. 2007;120:958–65.
21. Cornblath M, Hawdon JM, Williams AF, Aynsley-Green A, Ward-Platt MP, Schwartz R, Kalhan SC. Controversies regarding definition of neonatal hypoglycemia: suggested operational thresholds. Pediatrics. 2000;105:1141–5.
22. American Academy of Pediatrics Committee on Fetus and Newborn. Screening and management of postnatal glucose homeostasis in late preterm and term SGA and LGA/DM infants. Pediatrics. 2011;127:575–9.
23. Stanescu DL, Stanley CA. Advances in understanding the mechanism of transitional neonatal hypoglycemia and implications for management. Clin Perinatol. 2022;49:55–72.
24. Pezzati M, Barni S, Chiti G, Danesi G, Rubaltelli FF. Prolonged hyperinsulinemic hypoglycemia in a small for date preterm. Minerva Pediatr. 2003;55:79–82.
25. Polin R, Abman SH, Rowitch DH, Benitz W. Fetal and neonatal physiology. Elsevier; 2016.
26. MacDonald MG, Seshia MMK. Avery's neonatology: pathophysiology & management of the newborn. 7th ed. Lippincott Williams & Wilkins, a Wolters Kluwer Business; 2016.
27. Sunehag A, Ewald U, Gustafsson J. Extremely preterm infants (< 28 weeks) are capable of gluconeogenesis from glycerol on their first day of life. Pediatr Res. 1996;40:553–7.
28. Sunehag AL. The role of parenteral lipids in supporting gluconeogenesis in very premature infants. Pediatr Res. 2003;54:480–6.
29. Sunehag AL. Parenteral glycerol enhances gluconeogenesis in very premature infants. Pediatr Res. 2003;53:635–41.
30. Chacko SK, Sunehag AL. Gluconeogenesis continues in premature infants receiving total parenteral nutrition. Arch Dis Child Fetal Neonatal Ed. 2010;95:F413–8.
31. Limesand SW, Rozance PJ, Smith D, Hay WW Jr. Increased insulin sensitivity and maintenance of glucose utilization rates in fetal sheep with placental insufficiency and intrauterine growth restriction. Am J Physiol Endocrinol Metab. 2007;293:E1716–25.
32. Thorn SR, Brown LD, Rozance PJ, Hay WW Jr, Friedman JE. Increased hepatic glucose production in fetal sheep with intrauterine growth restriction is not suppressed by insulin. Diabetes. 2013;62:65–73.
33. Wesolowski SR, Hay WW Jr. Role of placental insufficiency and intrauterine growth restriction on the activation of fetal hepatic glucose production. Mol Cell Endocrinol. 2016;435:61–8.
34. Thornton PS, Stanley CA, De Leon DD, Harris D, Haymond MW, Hussain K, Levitsky LL, Murad MH, Rozance PJ, Simmons RA, Sperling MA, Weinstein DA, White NH, Wolfsdorf JI, Pediatric Endocrine Society. Recommendations from the pediatric endocrine society for evaluation and management of persistent hypoglycemia in neonates, infants, and children. J Pediatr. 2015;167:238–45.
35. Thorn SR, Rozance PJ, Brown LD, Hay WW Jr. The intrauterine growth restriction phenotype: fetal adaptations and potential implications for later life insulin resistance and diabetes. Semin Reprod Med. 2011;29:225–36.
36. Thorn SR, Regnault TR, Brown LD, Rozance PJ, Keng J, Roper M, Wilkening RB, Hay WW Jr, Friedman JE. Intrauterine growth restriction increases fetal hepatic gluconeogenic capacity and reduces messenger ribonucleic acid translation initiation and nutrient sensing in fetal liver and skeletal muscle. Endocrinology. 2009;150:3021–30.
37. Limesand SW, Rozance PJ. Fetal adaptations in insulin secretion result from high catecholamines during placental insufficiency. J Physiol. 2017;595:5103–13.

38. Limesand SW, Rozance PJ, Zerbe GO, Hutton JC, Hay WW Jr. Attenuated insulin release and storage in fetal sheep pancreatic islets with intrauterine growth restriction. Endocrinology. 2006;147:1488–97.
39. Chen X, Kelly AC, Yates DT, Macko AR, Lynch RM, Limesand SW. Islet adaptations in fetal sheep persist following chronic exposure to high norepinephrine. J Endocrinol. 2017;232:285–95.
40. Camacho LE, Chen X, Hay WW Jr, Limesand SW. Enhanced insulin secretion and insulin sensitivity in young lambs with placental insufficiency-induced intrauterine growth restriction. Am J Physiol Regul Integr Comp Physiol. 2017;313:R101–9.
41. Stanley CA, De Leon DD. Etiology of the neonatal Hypoglycemias. Adv Pediatr Infect Dis. 2024;71:119–34.
42. Stanley CA, Thornton PS, De Leon DD. New approaches to screening and management of neonatal hypoglycemia based on improved understanding of the molecular mechanism of hypoglycemia. Front Pediatr. 2023;11:1071206.

Chapter 5
Evidence for and Definitions of Normal and Abnormal Low Glucose Concentrations

David H. Adamkin

Introduction

Low blood glucose concentrations shortly after birth are the result of the delayed metabolic transition from maternal to endogenous neonatal sources of glucose. Neonatal hypoglycemia, frequently defined as <47 mg/dL or <2.6 mmol/L, may be found in up to 40% of neonates [1]. Up to 30% of infants are in the commonly accepted risk categories, making this risk of low blood glucose the most common reason for medical intervention in neonates outside of delivery room care [2]. The exact optimal plasma or blood glucose concentration thresholds for diagnosing and treating hypoglycemia are not yet supported by randomized clinical trials, nor is there an evidence based definition for neonatal hypoglycemia. More than 25 years ago, Cornblath, et al. noted that "The definition of clinically significant hypoglycemia remains one of the most confused and contentious issues in contemporary neonatology" [3]. Furthermore, a National Institutes of Health (NIH) workshop held in 2009 including pediatricians from the American Academy of Pediatrics (AAP) Committee for the Fetus and Newborn (COFN) reviewed published data regarding neonatal hypoglycemia, concluded that "there has been no substantial evidence-based progress in defining what constitutes clinically significant neonatal hypoglycemia. Monitoring for and prevention and treatment of neonatal hypoglycemia remain largely empirical" [4]. Subsequently, COFN published their statement in 2011 regarding neonatal hypoglycemia, Now some 14 years later the statement entitled Postnatal Glucose Homeostasis is under revision [5].

There still is no robust evidence to support most aspects of screening and management of neonates, or thresholds for blood or plasma glucose concentration thresholds for diagnosis and monitoring. The pathophysiology and mechanisms

D. H. Adamkin (✉)
Division of Neonatal Medicine, University of Louisville, Louisville, Kentucky, USA
e-mail: david.adamkin@louisville.edu

D. H. Adamkin, W. W. Hay, Jr. (eds.), *Disorders of Neonatal Glycemia*,
https://doi.org/10.1007/978-3-032-29094-6_5

relating to hypoglycemia and the brain are advancing but high certainty evidence on which to base clinical decision making remains controversial [6].

Definitions of hypoglycemia are based on epidemiologic, statistical, clinical, and neurophysiological studies [7, 8]. The statistical approach uses epidemiological studies with standard deviations or interquartiles [1, 9, 10]. It is important to note that a statistical norm is not a biological norm. Using these data a plasma glucose concentration of <47 mg/dL (2.6 mmol/L) corresponds to the tenth percentile for term infants during the first 48 h of life [1]. The clinical approach uses the glucose concentration seen when clinical symptoms first appear and when they disappear with treatment. The neurophysiological approach is based on the first abnormal sensory evoked potential following a blood glucose concentration of 13–45 mg/dL [11].

The confusion regarding a definition of neonatal hypoglycemia becomes clear when examining the various glucose concentration thresholds from diverse health organizations [12, 13]. Several currently used algorithms for diagnosing and treating hypoglycemia in term infants are summarized here:

The British Association of Paediatric Medicine (BAPM) uses a single blood glucose value of <2.5 mmol/L (45 mg/dL) over the first 48 h of life in a neonate with abnormal clinical signs [14]. They also use a blood glucose concentration of <2.0 mmol/L (36 mg/dL) that is persistent at the next measurement in an asymptomatic infant with a risk factor for hypoglycemia [14]. They define severe hypoglycemia at any time as a blood glucose concentration <1.0 mmol/L (18 mg/dL).

The American Academy of Pediatrics (AAP 2011) guidance in high-risk neonates uses a threshold for significant neonatal hypoglycemia in a symptomatic infant a blood glucose concentration <40 mg/dL (2.2 mmol/L) [5]. The blood glucose concentration <40 mg/dL (2.2 mmol/L) in an asymptomatic infant in the first hours after birth. From 4–24 h, they define significant hypoglycemia as a blood glucose concentration <45 mg/dL in an asymptomatic infant [5].

The Pediatric Endocrine Society (PES) from the United States, primarily concerned in finding neonates with suspected congenital hyperinsulinemic hypoglycemia, have proposed that a plasma glucose <70 mg/dL (3.9 mmol/L) should be treated [15]. For high risk neonates without suspected metabolic hypoglycemic disorders and aged under 48 h, their threshold plasma glucose concentration is <50 mg/dL (2.8 mmol/L). For neonates who are >48 h old, their threshold is a plasma glucose concentration <60 mg/dL (3.3 mmol/L) [15]. Table 5.1 offers a comparison between the initial AAP guidance and the PES.

Table 5.1 Comparison of the AAP and PES screening glucose concentration threshold values from 2012

	0–4 h[a]	4–24 h	24–48 h	>48 h
AAP[b]	<25–40 mg/dL	<35–45 mg/dL	<45 mg/dL	>60 mg/dL
PES	<50 mg/dL	<50 mg/dL	<50 mg/dL	>60 mg/dL

[a]The 0–4 h period includes the normal postnatal glucose nadir. Asymptomatic infants with low glucose values in this period do not require treatment other than feeding unless glucose concentrations that remain low for at least 4 h of life persist

[b]Any symptomatic infant with glucose concentration <40 mg/dL should receive IV dextrose

The World Health Organization (WHO) guidance for the newborn and young infant is to treat blood glucose concentrations of <2.2 mmol/L (40 mg/dL) [16]. Different thresholds may be applicable in infants at risk of hyperinsulinism or extending beyond the first 48 h after birth.

Postnatal Glucose Homeostasis and Transitional Neonatal Hypoglycemia

At birth the infant's blood glucose concentration is about 70% of the maternal level. It falls rapidly to a nadir by 1 h to a value as low as 20–25 mg/dL [17]. The nadir and these lower levels the first hours of life are prevalent in healthy neonates and are seen in all mammalian newborns. These levels are transient and begin to rise over the first hours and days of life. These lower levels during transition are considered to be part of the normal adaptation to postnatal life that helps establish postnatal glucose homeostasis [17–19]. Are there advantages to having a lower blood glucose concentration for the first 2 days of life? A decrease in glucose concentration soon after birth is essential to stimulate physiological processes that are required for postnatal survival, including promoting glucose production through gluconeogenesis and glycogenolysis [20] Additionally, the decreased glucose concentration enhances oxidative fat metabolism, stimulates appetite, and may help adapt to fast-feed cycles [20]. However, persistently lower glucose concentrations might result from mechanisms that were vital for the fetus to allow maternal-to fetal glucose transport but are not reversed after birth [20]. These persistently lower levels may be associated with peripartum stress, (fetal distress, birth asphyxia, or low Apgar scores) and with low weight-for-length ratios consistent with fetal growth restriction [12, 13]. Perinatal stress itself may be associated with usually transient hyperinsulinemic hypoglycemia that can continue for several days but even up to several weeks [21, 22].

The PES examined transitional neonatal hypoglycemia over the first 48 h of life using a neuroendocrine approach focusing on the major metabolic fuel and hormonal responses to low blood glucose levels during this period [23]. They noted this transition was characterized by hyperinsulinemia, suppressed levels of ketones, and reduced hyperglycemic responses to glucagon and epinephrine [24–26]. This metabolic profile was consistent with a neurogenic response at a glucose level of 55–65 mg/dL in older children and adults and therefore was considered by the PES as the normal glucose concentration that they advocated for the newborn infant. The adult neurogenic response stabilizes glucose concentrations and protects the brain. A value below 50 mg/dL is associated with brain injury from neuroglycopenia in the adult. However, we still do not know the plasma glucose concentration for neuroglycopenia or intracellular energy failure due to glucose inadequacy in the newborn.

The least common varieties of neonatal hypoglycemia are those that are persistent and recurrent. The most common causes of persistent hypoglycemia in the newborn are hyperinsulinemic hypoglycemia of infancy and congenital hyperinsulinism

[13]. These inherited disorders involve abnormalities of the mechanisms of insulin secretion by the pancreatic beta cell [13]. The definition of these conditions include blood glucose concentrations from <1.0 mmol/L (18 mg/dL) at any time and persistent hypoglycemia at a blood glucose concentration of <2.0 mmol/L (36 mg/dL) on three or more repeated measurements in the first 48 h [15]. Also considered as persistent hypoglycemia are those conditions occurring outside of the window of transitional newborn hypoglycemia (48–72 h) hours with higher normative values before assigning these as severe hypoglycemic levels, and any episode of low and persistent hypoglycemia requiring intravenous glucose for management [15, 29].

Clinical Studies and Low Glucose Levels

Clinical aspects of neonatal hypoglycemia include a wide variety of disorders and pathogeneses, with the common factor being the low blood glucose concentration. The incidence of neonatal hypoglycemia in a given population depends on the degree of risk, the timing of the screening, human milk feeding or formula, and above all the definition of hypoglycemia. Also, the use of continuous interstitial monitoring will increasingly identify low glucose concentrations that were not detected with intermittent glucose testing [30].

Testing for hypoglycemia includes two older studies that laid the groundwork and one also related the low concentrations to short- term outcomes [31, 32]. The first study had 232 "low risk" infants among whom the onset of hypoglycemia occurred at a mean age of 3.4 h and the incidence was 8% for hypoglycemia defined as a level of <30 mg/dL for full term and <20 mg/dL for low-birthweight infants [31]. Using 40 mg/dL to define hypoglycemia the incidence was 21% for all infants included in the study [31]. The second was a large multicenter study from 1988 with 661 preterm infants with birthweight less than 1800 g that were in an early diet and short outcomes study but also had glucose monitoring performed [32]. Ten percent of these infants had at least one value of blood glucose less than 10 mg/dL (0.06 mmol/L), 28% had at least one value less than 30 mg/dL (1.6 mmol/L), and 66% had at least one value less than 45 mg/dL [32]. Another study included 514 infants >35 weeks gestation at risk for hypoglycemia including small for gestational age (SGA), large for gestational age (LGA), infants of diabetic mothers (IDMs), and late preterm (LPT) infants who were screened for hypoglycemia over the first 48 h of life [33]. Fifty one percent of these infants had at least one episode of plasma glucose concentration below the arbitrarily chosen threshold of 47 mg/dL and 19% had a plasma glucose <36 mg/dL [33].

The threshold of glucose concentration chosen to diagnose hypoglycemia and the number of screening labs performed will affect the number of cases of neonatal hypoglycemia that will be diagnosed [34]. Applying the thresholds used for the high risk newborns (SGA, LGA, IDM, LPT) will diagnose neonatal hypoglycemia in 6%–19% of asymptomatic newborns who do not have risk factors during the first

48 h of life [34]. Infants with these risk factors and are therefore screened have a 50% risk of being diagnosed with hypoglycemia [33].

The method used to measure glucose is important. Point of care testing greater variability than lab measures, blood concentrations are lower than serum, and venous concentrations are lower than arterial [35]. Continuous glucose monitoring (CGM) is increasingly used both clinically and for research. CGM measures interstitial glucose concentrations that are directly related to plasma concentrations and provides an average glucose concentration value every 5 min showing dynamic glucose concentration trends [35, 36]. CGM appears to be safe, even in ELBW infants and despite being designed to detect hyperglycemia with lower accuracy for hypoglycemia it does identify more episodes of hypoglycemia than intermittent blood sampling [36, 37]. Using real time CGM a randomized controlled trial and a cohort of at-risk infants from the Children with Hypoglycemia and their Later Development trial (CHYLD), 25% of hypoglycemic events captured by CGM were missed by intermittent testing [30, 38]. Using CGM real time in other studies has been shown to reduce the number of hypoglycemic events, and randomized clinical trials have reported more time in the target glucose range [36, 39].

The Glucose in Well Babies (GLOW) study determined postnatal glucose concentration changes in plasma simultaneously with interstitial glucose concentrations (CGM) [1]. Sixty-seven infants were studied, mostly breastfed and in their own homes. Previous reports on the patterns of blood glucose in hospitalized neonates right after birth have shown a prompt fall in plasma glucose concentration reaching a nadir between 30 and 90 min after birth, followed by a spontaneous rise regardless of feeding [40, 41]. The GLOW study reported the mean plasma glucose concentration between 1 and 4 h to be 57.6 and 59.4 mg/dL for the first 48 h. Mean glucose concentrations increased between 48 and 72 h to reach values similar to adults of 82.8 mg/dL [1]. The third centile measurement for day 4 was 59.4 mg/dL [1]. There was considerable variation in glucose concentrations within and between babies, suggesting that the metabolic transition is gradual over the first 4 postnatal days. These observations suggest plasma glucose concentrations in neonates soon after birth increase over 18 h following the normal nadir and then remain stable to 48 h (~60 mg/dL) before increasing to a new plateau by the fourth day (~90 mg/dL). Plasma glucose concentrations of 47 mg/dL approximated the tenth percentile for the range of plasma glucose concentrations in the first 48 h for these well infants with no risk factors and 39% of these infants had >1 episode below 47 mg/dL [34].

In the same GLOW study, CGM showed that half of the infants were "hypoglycemic" at some point during this 2–4 day period using the threshold chosen [34]. A comparison of the results from this study with recommendations from the British Association of Perinatal Medicine, the World Health Organization, the PES, and the AAP shows the majority of healthy newborns with no risk factors will have some plasma glucose concentrations defined as abnormal that could lead to treatment for hypoglycemia. Table 5.2 shows glucose concentrations for both plasma and CGM from the GLOW study [42].

In Table 5.2, the data suggest that many healthy infants have glucose concentrations below the internationally recommended thresholds for treatment of at-risk

Table 5.2 Percent of healthy no risk infants with glucose levels below recommended thresholds for treatment from four guidelines

Percent that would require treatment at different hours after birth					
PLASMA (%)/CGM (%)					
Hours	0–4	4–24	24–48	48–72	72–120
AAP	0/0	3/11	1/5	1/2	0/0
BAPM	5/7	4/16	2/5	3/2	0/0
WHO	18/38	24/63	13/33	10/30	1/9
PES	25/50	40/73	22/58	46/73	6/55

From Adamkin et al. [34], reproduced with permission from Elsevier

Table 5.3 Number of healthy vs "at-risk infants" with episodes of low plasma glucose concentrations

Thresholds, mg/dL (mmol/L)	Plasma glucose healthy infants	At-risk infants	Interstitial glucose (CGM) healthy infants	At-risk infants
<47 [2.6]	26/67	159/326	37/51	33/44
	39%	49%	68%	75%
<36 [2.0]	7/67	48/326	12/51	14/44
	10%	15%	23%	32%
<27 [1.5]	0/67	9/326	0/51	3/44
	0%	3%	0%	7%

From Adamkin et al. [34], reproduced with permission from Elsevier

infants derived from historical data in the CHYLD and the GLOW study. Apparently healthy early term infants born at <40 weeks gestation are more likely to have episodes of low glucose concentrations as shown in Table 5.2 [42]. Similar to late preterm infants who are identified as a risk category, the data suggest that healthy early term infants are more likely to have low plasma glucose concentrations than more mature infants [1] (Table 5.3).

The GLOW study also measured alternative fuels to explore the physiology of the complex physiological changes of glucose over time [1]. Alternate substrates to glucose include lactate, ketones, and amino acids [27–29, 43]. In hypoglycemic newborns ketones only become available on the second or third day while presumably protective levels of lactate (>1.8 mM in adults) were identified in most infants during the first 48 h of life. However, the lactate concentrations did not increase with hypoglycemia [28]. Lactate concentrations are higher in the first 12 h of life before decreasing to a steady state value by 48 h [44]. The GLOW study also showed that glucose provides 72%–84% of cerebral fuel, while lactate furnishes 25% on the first day and ketones (primarily beta-hydroxybutyrate) supplies 7% on the second and third day [28].

These alternative substrate measurements from the GLOW study allow calculations such as the sum of glucose and beta-hydroxybutyrate or glucose-to-lactate ratio, which may be helpful to understanding neonatal dysglycemia [43, 44]. Data from the GLOW study shows that metabolic transition of healthy newborns is supported by alternative fuels and is completed by 48–72 h after birth [43]. All low glucose concentrations are not equal [1, 28]. The postnatal age of the infant and the metabolic milieu are critical to understanding the likely causes and consequences of low blood glucose concentrations in normal and at risk neonates [1, 44].

Clinical Signs

Clinicians have focused on clinical signs that might indicate insufficient circulating glucose to help determine urgency in screening and making diagnoses of hypoglycemia and to determine whether an infant might have glucose concentrations low enough to be at risk of progressively more severe hypoglycemia and the potential for incurring poor neurodevelopmental outcomes [45–47]. The development of risk category assignment prior to delivery is focused on screening those who might be at risk for low glucose concentrations. However, even apparently healthy term infants have developed moderately low glucose concentrations and later suffered neurodevelopmental and cognitive deficiencies [4].

Severe symptoms include progressive hypotonia leading to apnea, lethargy, coma, and seizures. Infants with such symptoms and low glucose concentrations require urgent evaluation and intervention, as these signs indicate possible brain injury. Other symptoms that occur earlier are related to adrenalin secretion and include jitteriness, trembling, irritability alternating with lack of alerting response to stimulation, intermittent floppiness or apparent fatigue, pallor, and feeding poorly after initially feeding well [8].

There clearly is variability in the clinical signs and their interpretation as well as uncertainty about any correlations with causes and outcomes [45, 48]. Hoerman et al. in 2022 reported on videos of 145 term infants with various glucose concentrations reviewed by 10 experienced clinicians and found poor correlation between clinical signs observed and accuracy in determining the degree of hypoglycemia [49]. Both sensitivity and specificity lacked statistical significance among the observers [49]. This study raises the question as to whether clinicians should rely on assessments of clinical signs in at risk infants [45]. Infants with progressive signs of hypoglycemia and low glucose concentrations should be evaluated. However, individual differences in clinicians' assessments and the marked variability in the clinical signs themselves and the different outcomes related to highly variable glucose concentrations must be appreciated [45].

References

1. Harris DL, Wesson PI, Gamble GD, Harding JE. Glucose profiles in healthy term infants in the first 5 days: the glucose in well babies (GLOW) study. J Pediatr. 2020;223:34–41.
2. O'Brien M, Gilchrist C, Sadler L, Hegarty JE, Alsweiler JM. Infants eligible for neonatal hypoglycemia screening: a systemic review and retrospective observational cohort study. J Pediatr. 2023;177:1187–96.

3. Cornblath M, Hawdon JM, Williams AF, Aynsley-Green A, Ward-Platt MP, Schwartz R, Kalhan SC. Controversies regarding definition of neonatal hypoglycemia: suggested operational thresholds. Pediatrics. 2000;105:1141–5.
4. Hay WW, Raju TN, Higgins RD, Kalhan SC, Devaskar SU. Knowledge gaps and research needs for understanding and treating neonatal hypoglycemia: workshop report for Eunice Kennedy Shriver National Institute of Child Health and Human Development. J Pediatr. 2009;155:612–7.
5. Adamkin DH, Committee on fetus and newborn. postnatal glucose homeostasis in late preterm, and term infants. Pediatrics. 2011;127:575–9.
6. Harding JE, Alsweiler JM, Edwards TE, McKinlay CJ. Neonatal hypoglycemia. BMJ Med. 2024;3:e000544.
7. Roeper M, Hoermann H, Kummer S, Meissner T. Neonatal hypoglycemia: lack of evidence for a safe management. Front Endocrine. 2023;14:1179102.
8. Hubbard EM, Hay WW Jr. The term newborn: hypoglycemia. Clin Perinatol. 2021;48:665–79.
9. Wight NE, Academy of Breastfeeding Medicine. ABM clinical protocol #1: guidelines for glucose monitoring and treatment of hypoglycemia in term and late preterm neonates, revised 2021. Breastfeed Med. 2021;16:353–65.
10. Wight NE. Hypoglycemia in breasted neonates. Breastfeed Med. 2006;1:253–62.
11. Koh TH, Aynsley-Green A, Tarbit M, Eyre J. A neural dysfunction during hypoglycemia. Arch Dis Chil. 1988;63:1353–8.
12. Legace M, Tam W. Neonatal Dysglycemia: a review of dysglycemia in relation to brain health and neurodevelopment outcomes. Pediatr Res. 2024;96:1429–37.
13. Cromb D, Radomska M, Thalange N, Cawley P. Fifteen minute consultation and management of hypoglycemia in the term born infant. Arch Dis Child Educ Pract Ed. 2011;109:73–81.
14. Levene I, Wilkinson D. Identification and management of neonatal hypoglycemia in the full term infant (British Association of Perinatal Medicine Framework for Practice). Arch Dis Child Educ Pract Ed. 2019;104:29–32.
15. Thornton PS, Stanley CA, De Leon DD, Harris D, Haymond MW, Hussain K, Levitsky LL, Murad MH, Rozance PJ, Simmons RA, Sperling MA, Weinstein DA, White NH, Wolfsdorf JI, Pediatric Endocrine Society. Recommendations from the Pediatric Endocrine Society for evaluation and management of persistent hypoglycemia in neonates, infants, and children. J Pediatr. 2015;167:238–45.
16. World Health Organization (WHO). Pocket book of hospital care for children: guidelines for the management of common childhood illnesses. 2nd ed. Geneva: World Health Organization; 2013.
17. Srinvasan G, Pildes RS, Cattamachi G, Voora S, Lilien LD. Plasma glucose values in normal neonates: a new look. J Pediatr. 1986;109:114–7.
18. Heck LJ, Erenberg A. Serum glucose levels in term neonates during the first 48 hours of life. J Pediatr. 1987;110:119–22.
19. Adamkin DH. Update on neonatal hypoglycemia. Arch Perinatal Med. 2005;11:13–5.
20. Rozance PJ, Hay WW Jr. Neonatal hypoglycemia—answers but more questions. J Pediatr. 2012;16:775–6.
21. Collins JE, Leonard JV, Teale D, Marks V, Williams DM, Kennedy CR, Hall MA. Hyperinsulinemic hypoglycemia in small for dates babies. Arch Dis Child. 1990;65:1118–20.
22. Hoe FM, Thornton PS, Wanner LA, Steinkrauss I, Simmons RA, Stanley CA. Clinical features and insulin regulation in infants with a syndrome of prolonged neonatal hyperinsulinism. J Pediatr. 2006;148:207–12.
23. Stanley CA, Rozance PJ, De Leon DD, Harris D, Haymond MW, Hussain K, Levitsky LL, Murad MH, Simmons RA, Sperling MA, Weinstein DA, White NH, Wolfsdorf JI. Re-evaluating "transitional neonatal hypoglycemia": mechanism and implications for management. J Pedatr. 2015;166:1520–5.
24. Hawdon JM, Ward Platt MP, Aynsley Green A. Pattern of metabolic adaptation for preterm and term infants in the first neonatal week. Arch Dis Child. 1992;67:357–65.

25. Desmond MM, Hild JR, Gast JH. The glycemic response of the newborn infant to epinephrine administration: a preliminary report. J Pediatr. 1950;37:341–50.
26. Stanley CA, Anday EK, Baker I, Delivoria-Papadopolous M. Metabolic fuel and hormone responses to fasting in newborn infants. Pediatrics. 1979;64:613–9.
27. Harris DL, Weston PI, Harding JE. Lactate, rather than ketones, may provide alternative cerebral fuel in hypoglycemic newborns. Arch Dis Child Did Fetal Neonatal Ed. 2015;100:F161–4.
28. Harris DL, Weston PI, Harding JE. Alternative fuels in the first five days in healthy term infants: the glucose in well babies (GLOW) study. J Pediatr. 2021;231:81–6.
29. Narvey MR, Marks SD. The screening and management of newborns at risk for low blood glucose. Paediatr Child Health. 2019;24:536–44.
30. McKinlay CJ, Alsweiler JM, Ansell JM, Anstice NS, Chase JG, Gamble GD, Harris DL, Jacobs RJ, Jiang Y, Paudel N, Signal M, Thompson B, Wouldes TA, Yu TY, Harding JE, CHYLD Study Group. Neonatal glycemia and neurodevelopmental outcomes at 2 years. NEJM. 2015;373:1507–18.
31. Diwakar KK, Sasidhar MV. Plasma glucose levels in term infants who are appropriate size for gestation and exclusively breast fed. Arch Dis Child. 2002;87:F46–8.
32. Lucas A, Morley R, Cole TJ. Adverse neurodevelopment outcome of moderate neonatal hypoglycemia. Br Med J. 1988;297:1304–8.
33. Harris DI, Weston P, Harding JR. Incidence of neonatal hypoglycemia in babies identified as at risk. J Pediatr. 2012;161:787–91.
34. Adamkin DH. Low blood sugar levels in the newborn infant: do changing goal posts matter? Semin Fetal Neonatal Med. 2021;26:101202.
35. Beardsall K. Measurement of glucose levels in the newborn. Early Hum Dev. 2010;86:263–7.
36. Beardsall K, Vanhaesebrouck S, Ogilvy-Stuart AL, Vanhole C, VanWeissenbruch M, Midgley P, Thio M, Cornette L, Ossuetta I, Palmer CR, Iglesias I, de Jong M, Gill B, de Zegher F, Dunger DB. Validation of the continuous glucose monitoring sensor in preterm infants. Arch Dis Child Fetal Neonatal Ed. 2013;98:F136–40.
37. Galderisi A, Facchinetti A, Steil GM, Ortiz-Rubio P, Cavallin F, Tamborlane WV, Baraldi E, Cobelli C, Trevisanuto D. Continuous glucose monitoring in very preterm infants: a randomized trial. Pediatrics. 2017;140:e20171162.
38. Uetwiller F, Chemin A, Bonnemaison E, Favrais G, Saliba E, Labarthe F. Real time continuous glucose monitoring reduces the duration of hypoglycemia episodes: a randomized control trial in very low birth weight neonates. PLoS One. 2015;10:e0116255.
39. Beardsall K, Thomson L, Guy C, Iglesias-Platas I, van Weissenbruch MM, Bond S, Allison A, Kim S, Petrou S, Pantaleo B, Hovorka R, Dunger D, REACT collaborative. Real time continuous glucose monitoring in preterm infants: an international open-label, randomized controlled trial. Lancet Child Adolesc Health. 2021;5:265–73.
40. Cornblath M, Reisner SH. Blood glucose in the neonate and its clinical significance. NEJM. 1965;273:378–81.
41. Kaiser JR, Bai S, Rozance PJ. Newborn plasma glucose concentration nadirs by gestational age group. Neonatology. 2018;113:353–9.
42. Barrington K. Let it Glow. Normal blood sugar profiles in newborn infants. Neonatal Research 6 May 2020 p 1–6. Available from https://neonatalresearch.org/2020/05/06/let-it-glow-normal-blood-sugar-profiles-in-newborn-infants/. Accessed 25 January 2021
43. Stanley CA, Weston PJ, Harris DL, De León DD, Harding JE. Role of beta-hydroxybutyrate measurement in the evaluation of plasma glucose concentrations in newborn infants. Arch Dis Child Fetal Neonatal Ed. 2024;109:580–5.
44. Galderisi A, Tordin M, Suppiej A, Cainelli E, Baraldi E, Trevisanuto D. Glucose-to-lactate ratio and neurodevelopment in infants with hypoxic ischemic encephalopathy: an observational study. Eur J Pediatr. 2023;182:837–44.
45. Hay WW Jr. Symptomatic or asymptomatic neonatal hypoglycemia-can one tell the difference? J Pediatr. 2022;245:7–9.

46. Adamkin DH. Metabolic screening and postnatal glucose homeostasis in the newborn. Pediatr Clin N Am. 2015;62:385–409.
47. Alkaly AL, Flores-Sarnat L, Sarnat HB, Farber SJ, Simmons CF. Plasma glucose concentrations in profound neonatal hypoglycemia. Clin Pediatr (Phila). 2006;45:550–8.
48. Cornblath M, Ichord R. Hypoglycemia in the neonate. Semin Perinatol. 2000;24:136–49.
49. Hoerman H, Mokwa A, Roeper M, Dafsari RS, Koestner F, Habenbeck C, Mayatepek E, Kummer S, Meissner T. Reliability and observer dependence of signs of neonatal hypoglycemia. J Pediatr. 2022;245:22–29.e2.

Chapter 6
Guidelines for Diagnosing Acute Neonatal Hypoglycemia; Searching for Neonatal Neuroglycopenia

David H. Adamkin

Introduction

Neuroglycopenia describes a state of metabolic imbalance caused by low rates of glycolysis that leads to a series of cellular events that impair function and cause injury. This series of events if not reversed may ultimately lead to cell necrosis [1, 2]. Neuroglycopenia mainly affects neurons, although glial cells may be susceptible to injury when hypoglycemia is combined with hypoxia [3]. Hypoglycemia induced apoptosis also has been reported in immature oligodendrocytes [4]. There are no clinical devices that can detect and monitor the initiation and progression of neuroglycopenia. As cell injury progresses, exogenous glucose may worsen cell injury. When NAD+ is depleted during hypoglycemia, reperfused glucose is shunted through the hexose monophosphate pathway, generating NADPH and more superoxide [5]. Superoxide can cause cellular injury and in animal models the rate of superoxide production is proportional to blood glucose levels after insulin induced hypoglycemia. The phenomenon of glucose reperfusion injury could explain why apparently brief and mild episodes of neonatal hypoglycemia have been associated with reduced educational achievement later in the affected infant's life [6].

Identifying a safe lower concentration of glucose and the duration of neonatal hypoglycemia has proved challenging in those infants who are receiving treatment [7]. Glucose reperfusion injury raises the question, to what extent are long term cognitive deficits after severe or recurrent hypoglycemia are only caused by hypoglycemia or the interventions the infants receive [8, 9]. For example, a prospective cohort of 477 infants born at risk of hypoglycemia, those who developed

D. H. Adamkin (✉)
Division of Neonatal Medicine, University of Louisville, Louisville, Kentucky, USA
e-mail: david.adamkin@louisville.edu

D. H. Adamkin, W. W. Hay, Jr. (eds.), *Disorders of Neonatal Glycemia*,
https://doi.org/10.1007/978-3-032-29094-6_6

neurosensory impairment at age 2 and 4.5 years were treated with higher and more rapid infusions of intravenous dextrose to increase blood concentrations of glucose that were below a threshold value of 47 mg/d [9, 10].

Neurodevelopmental Approach

A neurodevelopmental approach is aimed at finding the critical threshold of plasma glucose that is associated with brain injury thereby defining where "neuroglycopenia" occurs in the newborn. Neuroglycopenia in the adult occurs at a plasma glucose concentration threshold of <50 mg/dL. At levels between 55 and 65 mg/dL of plasma glucose the newborn infant, like the adult, demonstrates neuroendocrine and hormonal responses consistent with a neurogenic response [11]. This search for neonatal neuroglycopenia was profoundly influenced by a multicenter nutrition study from the United Kingdom published in 1988 (Fig. 6.1) [12].

The investigators concluded that 47 mg/dL represented a blood glucose concentration that could be associated with neuroglycopenia in the newborn [12]. The critical level of 47 mg/dL, still widely used today, came from this study. This multicenter trial included 661 preterm infants <1850 g at birth. Therefore, the study did not include late preterm or term infants with risk factors that are in the guidelines that are followed today. The study collected plasma glucose concentrations initially drawn daily, and then weekly until discharge. The primary purpose of this nutrition study was to determine the effect of early diet (human milk vs formula) on developmental outcomes at 18 months of age. The plasma glucose data revealed the

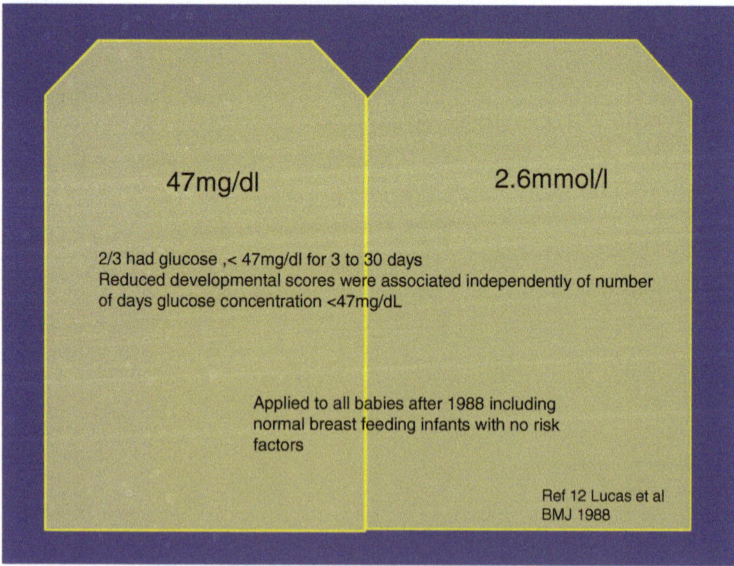

Fig. 6.1 Critical level of glucose 1998

number of days with "moderate hypoglycemia" (<47 mg/dL) correlated with reduced scores for mental and motor development at 18 months of age [12]. Many of the infants had plasma glucose levels <20 mg/dL for as long as 3–7 days prior to intervention since hypoglycemia was not a primary variable. At follow-up 7 years later, a letter to the journal written by the authors suggested this observational approach, assigning 47 mg/dL as a critical level, was problematic and that a randomized clinical trial like the nutrition study itself would be more valid [13]. Furthermore, these children at follow up at 7 years of age, had improved outcome vs their 18 months evaluation [12].

The value of <47 mg/dL from preterm infants <32 weeks in 1988 became the standard critical lower glucose concentration threshold for even term appropriate for gestational age (AGA) infants [14]. A prospective study 25 years later, also from the UK, included similar gestational infants (<32 weeks) [15]. Blood glucose concentrations were measured during the first 10 days of life among 47 of 566 babies (8%) who had a blood glucose <47 mg/dL on at least three of the first 10 days [15]. All were matched with controls who never had a blood glucose <47 mg/dL. No differences were found in developmental progress at 5 years of age [15]. Remarkably, 81% of the original cohort were matched again with controls at 15 years of age and the groups were almost identical in full scale IQ and other measures of outcome [16] The inclusion of children who had a level <47 mg/dL for >4 days and another group with levels <37 mg/dL on three different days did not alter the results [16].

A more recent controversy is whether low blood glucose concentrations during transitional hypoglycemia during the first hours of life may be associated with adverse neurodevelopment. This poses the question, should strategies be studied to modify these lower glucose concentrations in the first hours to improve outcomes in childhood. In a unique study from the State of Arkansas, 1400 infants who had transitional hypoglycemia, defined as at least a single glucose concentration <45 mg/dL, were tested at 10 years of age for academic achievement. On the basis of fourth grade school examinations the study linked a single episode of neonatal blood glucose concentration of <45 mg/dL that had resolved with the next glucose concentration measured by 3 h of age with a 50% reduction in achieving proficiency in literacy or numeracy (Fig. 6.2) [6]. This group of patients represented all of the deliveries during a calendar year, so most of the study patients were late preterm and term infants [6]. The cut-off values for transitional hypoglycemia were <30, <40, and <45 mg/dL, respectively. These low glucose concentrations were followed by a second concentration above those cut-offs. It is not certain if the low glucose group had only this one episode of hypoglycemia since no values were reported after the "normalization" of the second concentration.

What is the link between transitional hypoglycemia and subsequent poor academic performance? Is it possible that a brief period of low blood glucose may be a marker for other perinatal issues or adverse factors including events during intrauterine development. There is interest in learning more about these relationships and if strategies should be explored to increase glucose concentrations in the first hours of life. Current guidelines recommend screening only for newborns who are symptomatic or at risk of developing hypoglycemia. The Arkansas study suggests

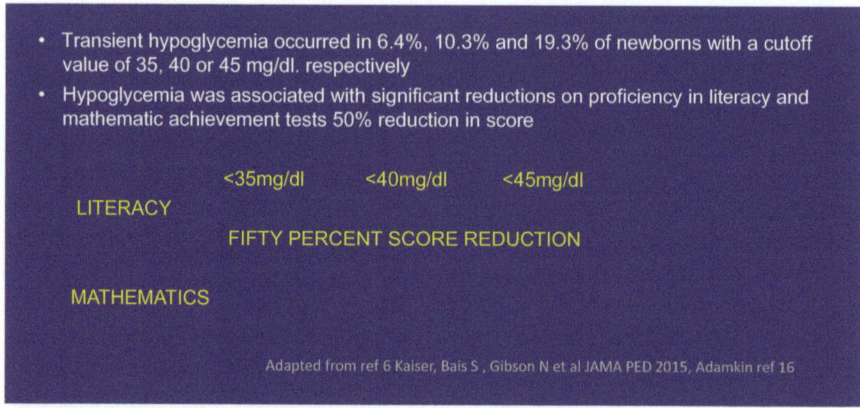

Fig. 6.2 Association between transient newborn hypoglycemia and fourth grade achievement test proficiency

that we should consider universal screening [14]. Screening is only justified when you can impact outcome with the result of the screen. The brief period of "hypoglycemia" in this study was diagnosed at 90 min of age, but the actual result was only available 30 min after that [6]. The second measurement showing resolution above one of the chosen three thresholds (<30, <40, <45 mg/dL) came 70 min after the first screen, or at 3 h of age. It is unlikely that any intervention after the results are known could shorten the exposure to this brief period of low blood glucose [16]. Is mild transitional hypoglycemia a cause of abnormal neurodevelopment or does it represent a marker of physiological instability associated with adverse development [16]? More research will be necessary to answer this question.

A more recent study also linked transitional neonatal hypoglycemia and neurodevelopment in mid childhood [17]. This cohort study of 140 children, aged 7–11 years had at least one blood glucose measurement of <30 mg/dL in the nursery and had follow-up neurodevelopmental testing at ~9 years [17]. These children were compared with those in which all measured glucose levels were above 30 mg/dL during postnatal blood glucose screening starting on the first day of life [17]. Children with what they defined as severe neonatal hypoglycemia (<30 mg/dL) had a 4.8 points lower mean full-scale IQ than controls. They had a 4.9 fold increased odds of abnormal fine motor function, and a 5.3 fold increased odds of abnormal visual motor integration [17]. Controls were recruited by telephone and email vs the list of 70 eligible low glucose patients. Controls were matched to the study group for sex, birth weight, gestational age, and socioeconomic status [18]. The first blood glucose measurement was performed within 2 h of life with a median of 1–1.5 h in the low glucose group. The lowest blood glucose occurred in 61% within the first 2 h, in ~28% between 2–12 h of age, 7% between 12–24 h, and ~6% >24 h [17]. Therefore, almost 40% of the low glucose study patients developed their low glucose concentrations outside of the first hours of life. In the low blood glucose group mean (SD) of lowest blood glucose was 22.3 (5.2) mg/dL [17]. In the controls the mean (SD) of lowest glucose concentrations was 48.1 (12.1) mg/dL [17]. Thirty seven controls (~53%) had at least one glucose measurement between 31 and 45 mg/dL. The retrospective design may compromise accuracy with glucose concentrations. The wide range of concentrations as well as the overlap is concerning in assigning outcomes. Like the Arkansas study there may also be confounders not matched between the groups that could have played a role in the outcome. Finally, the range of hours of the low glucose measurements is not typical of transitional hypoglycemia. The idea of altering transitional hypoglycemia by treatments to raise the blood glucose concentration is not yet supported with strong evidence.

The natural history of transitional neonatal hypoglycemia and its effects on long term neurodevelopmental outcomes are not well understood [19, 20]. In fact there is no direct evidence from randomized controlled trials that treatment of neonatal hypoglycemia improves long term neurodevelopmental outcome [21]. Thresholds to define neonatal hypoglycemia vary widely because of the uncertainty where blood glucose concentrations are associated with neuroglycopenia. Among different guidelines, operational thresholds for treatment range from 36 mg/L to 50 mg/dL [22]. In a large randomized controlled trial, 689 otherwise healthy >35 week gestational age "at risk" infants were enrolled in a study treating moderate hypoglycemia. The goal was to balance a treatment of a lower threshold without risking adverse consequences, while avoiding overutilization of health care resources (Fig. 6.3) [23].

The study compared traditional treatment to keep glucose concentrations >47 mg/dL vs treatment at a lower threshold of 36 mg/dL [23]. This HypoEXIT trial allowed for <0.5 SD below the mean cut-off for noninferiority (1 SD is considered normal) regarding cognitive and psychomotor outcomes at 18 months measured by the Bayley Scales of Infant and Toddler Development (BSID111). The mean glucose was 57 mg/dL in the lower threshold group and 61 mg/dL in the traditionally treated group [22]. The pre-specified inferiority limit was not crossed. Therefore, the lower threshold was non-inferior to the traditional threshold for neurodevelopmental outcome at age 18 months [23]. The problem with studies like this, even

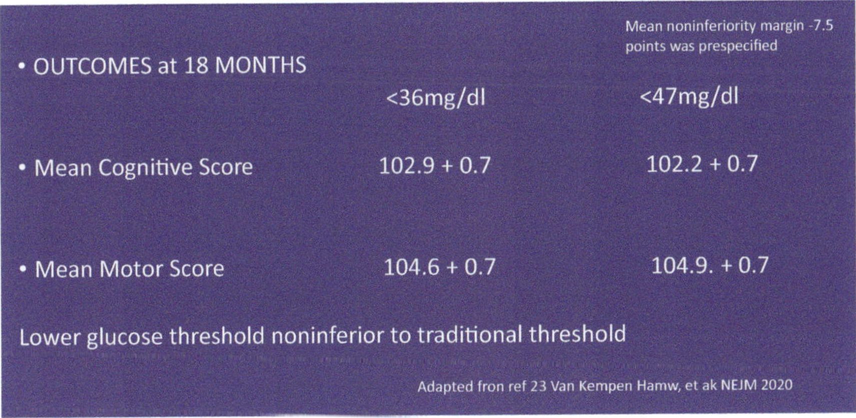

Fig. 6.3 Lower treatment threshold for neonatal hypoglycemia

with many subjects, is the age at follow up. Evaluations at 18 months for longer term outcomes might be too early to predict school age performance. However, it does show the confusion with determining glucose concentration thresholds at which neuroglycopenia might occur.

The Children with Hypoglycemia and their Later Development studies (CHYLD) continue to add information about the effects of neonatal hypoglycemia on developmental outcomes. The studies use the level of <47 mg/dL as the threshold for hypoglycemia [16]. In 2015 the investigators reported on over 600 late preterm and term infants at-risk for hypoglycemia [10]. The studies also included CGM recording a glucose level every 5 min [10]. The infants were treated aggressively to maintain plasma glucose >47 mg/dL. Using the CGM they observed long and undetected periods of glucose concentrations below the threshold detected only on CGM but missed on intermittent sampling [10]. More than half of the infants at risk were diagnosed with hypoglycemia and ~25% had undetected hypoglycemia using intermittent sampling and 25% of these episodes that were only detected with CGM lasted greater than 5 h [10]. Follow-up at age 2 years was reported among groupings, including a reference group who never had hypoglycemia, any episode of hypoglycemia, >3 days of hypoglycemia, or severe hypoglycemia defined as <36 mg/dL [10]. There was no association between neonatal hypoglycemia and neurodevelopmental outcome at 2 years of age [10]. Even those with undetected episodes of hypoglycemia on CGM showed no differences in neurosensory impairment or processing difficulty relative to controls. However, at 4.5 years of age, the follow up demonstrated executive function difficulties in those infants suffering more than one episode of hypoglycemia found only with CGM [27].

A prospective cohort study from the CHYLD group reported that of 477 moderate to late preterm and term infants born with risk factors and had a level of <47 mg/dL (2.6 mmol/L) were more likely to have executive dysfunction (adjusted risk ratio 2.32, 95% CI 1.17–4.49) and poor visual function (adjusted risk ratio 3.67, 95% CI 1.15–11.69) at age 4.5 years [8]. However, these poorer outcomes did not persist at age 9–10 years among 480 children (adjusted risk ratio 0.9, 95% CI 0.78–1.15) [7]. The at-risk children with no demonstration of hypoglycemia had similarly high rates of poor educational achievement as those who were hypoglycemic [9]. Again the possibility that being at risk for a lower glucose concentration might contribute independently to outcomes [9], supporting the problem with placing too much meaning on a single glucose concentration. Consistent with this discussion is that a large, randomized trial of dextrose gel prophylaxis, the treatment reduced the incidence of hypoglycemia but did not reduce the risk of adverse outcomes [24, 25]. This is despite the hypoglycemia being associated with poorer neurodevelopment in the same participant cohort [26].

In retrospective observational studies, either none of the risk factors used for screening was associated with hypoglycemia or only the use of insulin with maternal gestational diabetes was predictive of low blood glucose [28, 29]. The frequency of hypoglycemia in infants with risk factors was not significantly increased. Perhaps these infants are more sensitive to the effects of the hypoglycemia on neurodevelopment than infants with no risk factors [26].

The reason for screening and treatment is to prevent brain injury from neonatal hypoglycemia. Low quality evidence supports that severe, prolonged hypoglycemia can be responsible for neurological injury and even death, although these outcomes are highly variable as many infants who had such outcomes also had comorbid conditions which may themselves have influenced the outcomes [30–32]. Clearly, in children with persistent hyperinsulinemia, severe and recurrent hypoglycemia, poor neurological outcomes are much more common, and are seen even more often in those children who had suffered more severe levels of hypoglycemia with seizures, flaccid hypotonia with coma, and delays in detection and treatment [31]. A meta-analysis of six older studies that were considered of lower quality included 1657 children reported similar odds of impairment from age 2–5 years in children who did and did not have neonatal hypoglycemia [19]. The ranges of thresholds for diagnosing hypoglycemia ranged from 1.1 mmol/L (~20 mg/dL) to 2.6 mmol/L (47 mg/dL); odds ratio 1.16, 95% confidence interval 0.86–1.57 [19]. Two other studies of 54 children reported that those who had neonatal hypoglycemia were more likely to have neurodevelopmental impairment when assessed at age 6–11 years (two studies, 54 children; odds ratio 3.62, 1.05–12.42). This indicates that later follow up is likely necessary to diagnose any linkage between early neonatal hypoglycemia for the level selected in the study and neurodevelopmental outcome. However, the numbers of infants included in such studies are small, making firm conclusions from these studies relatively elusive.

More recent evidence suggests that even mild, brief, and asymptomatic hypoglycemia could be associated with poorer outcome. This evidence is conflicting and causal mechanisms are unclear [9]. A large secondary analysis from a randomized trial published in 2022 included 1194 late preterm and term infants with risk factors who were screened and treated if plasma glucose was <47 mg/dL [26]. This glucose concentration threshold was associated with poorer neurodevelopment at age 2 years (adjusted risk ratio 1.28, 95% CI 1.01–1.60), and this risk was even greater with severe hypoglycemia (<36 mg/dL; adjusted risk ratio 1.68, 1.2–2.36) [26]. Another large population study also reported an increased risk of any neurological or neurodevelopmental impairment with threshold glucose concentration of <40 mg/dL for children aged 2–6 years (adjusted risk ratio 1.48, 1.17–1.88) [33].

Evidence from these two randomized controlled trials that come to different conclusions show how limiting and conflicting the studies can be [9]. Two trials reported on the use of dextrose gel prophylactically to prevent transitional "hypoglycemia" [34, 35]. Both report that the infants randomized to receive the gel had a lower risk of a plasma glucose <47 mg/dL (relative risk 0.79, 95% CI 0.64–0.98, n = 416 and 0.88, 0.80–0.98, n = 2149). At the age of 2 years both studies found no differences in the risk of neurosensory impairment among the treated versus the control infants which was the main outcome [25, 36]. The first trial reported a trend towards improved secondary outcomes including language, motor, and executive function in the dextrose gel group [36]. However, the second trial reported worse language, motor, and cognitive function in the dextrose gel group [25].

How do we explain these conflicting outcomes? Differences in the characteristics of the infants, the duration and severity of the hypoglycemia, or availability of alternative brain substrates have not been measured in these studies and could be responsible. Infants with comorbid conditions like hypoxia-ischemia also could confound results [10, 24]. Furthermore, infants who are defined as "at risk" for neonatal hypoglycemia are diagnosed as such at birth, which might indicate that their adverse outcomes are the result of neurological injuries that occurred before birth, making post-birth hypoglycemia a marker and not a cause of such in utero injuries. This also might explain why it has been difficult to show that preventions and treatments of early and usually transient (transitional) neonatal hypoglycemia are not convincingly successful.

Screening and Monitoring

Neonatal hypoglycemia is commonly asymptomatic, unless severe, and as previously reviewed, clinical assessment has poor sensitivity and specificity for detecting low blood glucose levels [37, 38]. Therefore guidance from organizations such as the AAP and the PES recommends linking risk factors to determine which asymptomatic infants to screen [9]. Also, the thresholds for diagnosing hypoglycemia in asymptomatic infants differ among the guidelines [39]. Screening should identify a condition for which the natural course and history of the condition is understood. A reliable test for diagnosing neuroglycopenia would need to be based on studies of treatments that have reliably and with scientific validity improved outcomes [14]. This also means that the treatments have been shown to improve outcomes at a presymptomatic stage compared with usual care, and that the overall benefits of screening outweigh the harm [40, 41].

Measurement of glucose concentrations in plasma by laboratory chemical analyzers or in whole blood by blood gas analyzers are the accepted standards to measure plasma or whole blood glucose concentrations. CGM offers the possibility of adjusting treatment in real time to improve glucose stability, avoid undetected episodes of hypoglycemia, and reduce pain stress by decreasing the number of heel pricks for blood glucose testing. However, measuring tissue glucose in neonates is difficult because of the low operating range required and the rapidly changing blood glucose concentrations which make calibration of these instruments difficult [9, 42].

Subcutaneous sensors measure electric current generated by the oxidation of glucose from the interstitial fluid when voltage is applied However, none of the current systems has been designed for neonates [9]. Accuracy of these devices may be poor, especially at low glucose concentrations where 95% limits of agreement can exceed 1 mmol/L or 18 mg/dL [43, 44]. Thus one potential use for CGM is to screen and guide frequency of blood glucose testing. One study in very low birthweight infants found that blood glucose measurements guided by CGM reduced the number of capillary blood tests by 25% [45].

There also have been no studies comparing long term neurodevelopmental outcome of at-risk infants screened for neonatal hypoglycemia versus those not screened. However, screening infants at risk of hypoglycemia to maintain a blood glucose concentration of at least 47 mg/dL appears to preserve cognitive function compared to those who were screened but did not require treatment because they did not have hypoglycemia [42]. CGM suggests that infants with episodes of low glucose concentrations that were not detected by conventional blood testing and therefore were not treated were associated with reduced executive function in later childhood but were otherwise not different from infants monitored by CGM who did not have low glucose concentrations [46].

Management

The initial prevention and treatment of hypoglycemia is feeding and is dependent on what threshold clinical practices adopt as the baseline for intervention. Breastfeeding is prioritized but in the first days after birth breast milk volumes are modest and lactose and calorie content is low [47–49]. A prospective study including 62 healthy term infants showed an increase of blood glucose concentrations after breast feeding in the first 5 days after prolonged breast feeding (>30 min) and feeding from both breasts. This study observed little or no increase in blood glucose concentrations without prolonged feeding and feeding from both breasts [47]. Initiation of breastfeeding within the first hour of life has been a consistent recommendation. When breastfeeding is not possible within the first hour or two after birth, alternatives like pasteurized donor milk or formula can prevent delays in initial steps to prevent hypoglycemia [16]. The routine use of prophylactic dextrose gel with breastfeeding for infants with risk factors is not recommended because data do not support its effectiveness in improving neurodevelopmental outcomes [25]. A practical approach to feeding the infant at risk for or with transitional hypoglycemia is to encourage breastfeeding for longer periods and from both breasts, rather than expressing breast milk [16]. Caloric fortification is a strategy that some have used for those infants with a more persistent neonatal hypoglycemia and could be reasonable in SGA infants with IUGR and preterm infants who require extra calories for growth but perhaps not in other neonatal populations in whom the impact of early excessive caloric intake might have adverse effects on later growth of fat mass.

Dextrose gel is usually administered to infants with diagnosed hypoglycemia at a dose of 0.5 mL/kg of 40% dextrose gel (200 mg/kg), rubbed into the buccal mucosa, followed by a feed. In the Sugar Babies randomized trial including 242 infants compared with feeding alone, dextrose gel reduced the risk of treatment failure, intravenous treatment, and admission to the neonatal intensive care unit for treatment of hypoglycemia, while increasing successful breastfeeding [50]. Treatment can be repeated as needed, but most guidelines recommend an upper limit on the number of doses (usually two or three per episode of hypoglycemia, and a maximum of five or six doses in 48 h). It should be noted that this dextrose gel intervention did not impact neurodevelopment at 2 or 4.5 years of age [51].

If feeding and dextrose gel do not prevent or correct the hypoglycemia, then intravenous dextrose is the next step in treatment. Initial infusion rates of 3–5 mg/

kg/min are relatively standard. This rate is similar to neonatal glucose requirements that normally are produced endogenously. Additional increases in volume or concentration, or both are used as needed to maintain euglycemia in more severe cases. Greater uncertainty and some controversy surrounds the use of the "mini bolus" of 1–2 mL/kg of 10% dextrose. It is quick and easy to administer and achieves a prompt increase in blood glucose concentrations [52]. The controversy comes from the association between high and unstable glucose concentrations after bolus dextrose treatments of neonatal hypoglycemia and adverse neurodevelopmental outcomes [10]. Infants treated with intravenous dextrose, rather than dextrose gel, formula, or breast milk, are more likely to have high and unstable glucose concentrations [53]. Therefore, hypoglycemia and its treatment may have a "U-shaped" curve for risk of morbidity. A large before-and-after cohort study reported that a graded approach to both the use of the bolus and the rate of infusion, depending on severity of the hypoglycemia, improved stability of blood glucose concentration and shortened the length of stay in the NICU without changing the time to achieve a normal glucose concentration [54].

Conclusions

The search for neuroglycopenia in the late preterm and term neonate continues. Noninvasive screening tests and measurements from one touch screens of neuroendocrine metabolites may allow more accurate decision making to prevent injury. Exploring the role of neuroprotective substrates other than glucose to stabilize neuronal metabolism could open exciting possibilities in brain protection. Still more studies and randomized trials must examine early thresholds for decision making that have adequate and longer follow-up data to know the relationships between early low blood glucose concentrations and mediators of neuronal metabolism. The expansion and accuracy of CGM will aid in understanding the true variability of glucose metabolism and the relationship of glucose concentrations to biochemical and hormonal markers and clinical signs.

References

1. De Angelis LC, Brigati G, Polleri G, Malova M, Parodi A, Minghetti D, Rossi A, Massirio P, Traggiai C, Maghnie M, Ramenghi LA. Neonatal hypoglycemia and brain vulnerability. Front Endocrinol (Lausanne). 2021;12:634305.
2. Suh SW, Hamby AM, Swanson RA. Hypoglycemia, brain energetics, and hypoglycemic neuronal death. Glia. 2007;55:1280–6.
3. Lyons SA, Kettenmann H. Oligodendrocytes and microglia are selectively vulnerable to combined hypoxia and hypoglycemia injury in vitro. J Cereb Blood Flow Metab. 1998;18:521–30.
4. Yan H, Rivkees SA. Hypoglycemia influences oligodendrocyte development and myelin formation. Neurodevelopment. 2006;17:55–9.

5. Suh SW, Gum ET, Hamby AM, Chan PH, Swanson RA. Hypoglycemic neuronal death is triggered by glucose reperfusion and activation of neuronal NADPH oxidase. J Clin Invest. 2007;117:910–8.
6. Kaiser JR, Bai S, Gibson N, Holland G, Lin TM, Swearingen CJ, Mehl JK, ElHassan NO. Association between transient newborn hypoglycemia and fourth grade achievement test proficiency: a population based study. JAMA Pediatr. 2015;169:913–21.
7. Shah R, DWT D, Alsweiler JM, Brown GTL, Chase JG, Gamble GD, Harris DL, Keegan P, Nivins S, Wouldes TA, Thompson B, Turuwhenua J, Harding JE, McKinlay CJD, Children with Hypoglycaemia and their Later Development (CHYLD) Study Team. Association of neonatal hypoglycemia with academic performance in mid-childhood. JAMA. 2022;327:1158–70.
8. McKinlay CID, Alsweiler JM, Anstice NS, McKinlay CJD, Children with Hypoglycaemia and their Later Development (CHYLD) Study Team. Association of neonatal hypoglycemia with neurodevelopmental outcomes at 4.5 years. JAMA Pediatr. 2017;17:1972–83.
9. Harding JE, Alsweiler JM, Taygen EE, McKinlay CJD. Neonatal hypoglycemia. BMJ Med. 2024;3:3e000544.
10. McKinlay CJD, Alsweiler JM, Anstice NS, Chase JG, Gamble GD, Harris DL, Jacobs RJ, Jiang Y, Paudel N, Signal M, Thompson B, Wouldes TA, Yu TY, Harding JE, CHYLD Study Group. Neonatal glycemia and neurodevelopmental outcomes at 2 years. N Engl J Med. 2015;373:1507–18.
11. Stanley G, Rozance P, Thornton PS, De Leon DD, Harris D, Haymond MW, Hussain K, Levitsky LL, Murad MH, Simmons RA, Sperling MA, Weinstein DA, White NH, Wolfsdorf JI. Re-evaluating transitional neonatal hypoglycemia: mechanism and implications for management. J Pediatr. 2015;166:1520–5.e1.
12. Lucas A, Morley R, Cole TJ. Adverse neurodevelopmental outcome of moderate neonatal hypoglycaemia. Br Med J. 1988;297:1304–8.
13. Lucas A, Morley R. Outcome of neonatal hypoglycemia (letter). BMJ. 1999;318(7177):195.
14. Adamkin DH. Low blood sugar in the newborn infant: do changing goal posts matter? Semin Fetal and Neonatal Med. 2022;26(3):101202.
15. Tin W, Brumskill G, Kelly T, Fritz S. 5 year follow up of recurrent hypoglycemia in preterm infants. Pediatrics. 2012;130:1497–503.
16. Adamkin DH. Neonatal hypoglycemia. Semin Fetal and Neonatal Med. 2017;22:36–41.
17. Roeper M, Korner LM, Sobotka M, Mayatepek E, Kummer S, Meisner T. Transitional neonatal hypoglycemia and adverse neurodevelopment in Midchildhood. JAMA Netw Open. 2024;7:e243683.
18. Lampert T, Hoebel J, Kuntz B, Muters S, Kroll LE. Socioeconomic status and subjective social status measurement in KIGGS wave 2. J Healthy Monit. 2018;3:108–25.
19. Shah R, Harding J, Brown J, McKinlay C. Neonatal glycemia and neurodevelopmental outcomes: a systematic review and meta-analysis. Neonatology. 2019;115:116–26.
20. Horwitz J, Mardiros L, Musa A, Welch VA, Hodgson A, Narvey M, Ghazzawi A, Shea B, Saginur M. Scoping review of evidence for managing postnatal hypoglycemia. BMJ Open. 2022;12:e053047.
21. Edwards T, Liu G, Battlin M, Harris DL, Hegarty JE, Weston PJ, Harding JE. Oral dextrose gel for the treatment of hypoglycemia in newborn infants. Cochrane Database Sys Rev. 2022;3:3CD011027.
22. Thornton PS, Stanley CA, De Leon DD, Harris D, Haymond MW, Hussain K, Levitsky LL, Murad MH, Rozance PJ, Simmons RA, Sperling MA, Weinstein DA, White NH, Wolfsdorf JI, Pediatric Endocrine Society. Recommendations from the Pediatric Endocrine Society for evaluation and management of persistent hypoglycemia in neonates, infants, and children. J Pediatr. 2015;167:238–45.
23. van Kempen AAMW, Eskes PF, Nuytemans DHGM, van der Lee JH, Dijksman LM, van Veenendaal NR, van der Hulst FJPCM, Moonen RMJ, Zimmermann LJI, van 't Verlaat EP, van Dongen-van Baal M, Semmekrot BA, Stas HG, van Beek RHT, Vlietman JJ, Dijk PH, Termote JUM, de Jonge RCJ, de Mol AC, Huysman MWA, Kok JH, Offringa M, Boluyt N,

HypoEXIT Study Group. Lower versus traditional treatment for neonatal hypoglycemia. N Engl J Med. 2020;382:534–44.
24. Boluyt N, van Kempen A, Offringa M. Neurodevelopment after neonatal hypoglycemia a systematic review and design of an optimal future study. Pediatrics. 2006;117:2231–43.
25. Edwards T, Alsweiler JM, Crowther CA, Edlin R, Gamble GD, Hegarty JE, Lin L, McKinlay CJD, Rogers JA, Thompson B, Wouldes TA, Harding JE. Prophylactic oral dextrose gel and neurosensory impairment at 2 year follow up of participants in the hPOD randomized trial. JAMA. 2022;327:1149–57.
26. Edwards T, Alsweiler JM, Gamble GD, Griffith R, Lin L, McKinlay CJD, Rogers JA, Thompson B, Wouldes TA, Harding JE. Neurocognitive outcomes at age 2 years after neonatal hypoglycemia in a cohort of participants from the hPOD randomized trial. JAMA Netw Open. 2022;5:e22359.
27. Harris DI, Alsweiler JM, Ansell JM, Gamble GD, Thompson B, Wouldes TA, Yu TY, Harding JE, Children with Hypoglycaemia and their Later Development (CHYLD) Study Team. Outcomes at two years after dextrose gel treatment for neonatal hypoglycemia; follow up of a randomized controlled trial. J Pediatr. 2016;170:54–9.
28. Cummings CT, Ritter V, Le Blanc S, Sutton AG. Evaluation of risk factors and approach to screening for asymptomatic neonatal hypoglycemia. Neonatology. 2022;119:77–83.
29. Chen Y-S, Ho CH, Lin SJ, Tsai WH. Identifying additional risk factors for early asymptomatic neonatal hypoglycemia in term and late preterm babies. Pediatric Neonatology. 2022;63:625–32.
30. Anderson JM, Milner RD, Strich SJ. Effects of neonatal hypoglycemia on the nervous system: a pathological study. J Neurol Neurosurg Psychiatry. 1967;30:295–310.
31. Roeper M, Salimi Dafsari R, Hoerman H, Mayatepek E, Kummer S, Meissner T. Risk factors for adverse neurodevelopment in transient or persistent congenital hyperinsulinism. Front Endocrin (Lausanne). 2020;11:580642.
32. Montassir H, Maegaki Y, Ogura K, Kurozawa Y, Nagata I, Kanzaki S, Ohno K. Associated factors in neonatal hypoglycemic brain injury. Brain Dev. 2009;31:649–56.
33. Wickstron R, Skiold B, Peterson G, Stephansson O, Altman M. Moderate neonatal hypoglycemia and adverse neurologic development at 2–6 years of age. Eur J Epidemiol. 2018;33:1011–20.
34. Hegarty JE, Harding JE, Gamble GD, Crowther CA, Edlin R, Alsweiler JM. Prophylactic oral dextrose gel for newborn babies at risk of neonatal hypoglycemia: a randomized controlled dose finding trial (the pre-hPOD study). PLoS Med. 2016;18:e1003411.
35. Harding JE, Hegarty JE, Crowther CA, Edlin RP, Gamble GD, Alsweiler JM, hPOD Study Group. Evaluation of oral dextrose gel for prevention of neonatal hypoglycemia (hPOD) a multi-center, double blind randomized controlled trial. PLoS Med. 2021;18:e1003411.
36. Griffith R, Hegarty JE, Alsweiler JM, Gamble GD, May R, McKinlay CJD, Thompson B, Wouldes TA, Harding JE. Two year outcomes after dextrose gel prophylaxis for neonatal hypoglycemia. Arch Dis Child Fetal Neonatal Ed. 2021;106:278–85.
37. McKinlay CJD, Alsweiler JM, Bailey MJ, Cutfield WS, Rout A, Harding JE. A better taxonomy for neonatal hypoglycemia is needed. J Perinatol. 2021;41:1205–6.
38. Hoerman H, Mokwa, Roeper M, Salimi Dafsari R, Koestner F, Hagenbeck C, Mayatepek E, Kummer S, Meissner T. Reliability and observer dependence of signs of neonatal hypoglycemia. J Pediatr. 2022;245:22–9.
39. British Association of Perinatal Medicine (BAPM). Identification and management of neonatal hypoglycaemia in the full term infant: framework for practice. British Association of Perinatal Medicine; 2017. Available: https://hubble-live-assets.s3.amazonaws.com/bapm/file_asset/file/37/Identification_and_Management_of_Neonatal_Hypoglycaemia_in_the__full_term_infant_-_A_Framework_for_Practice_revised_Oct_2017.pdf.
40. Wilson JMG, Junger G. Principles and practice of screening for disease. WHO Chron. 1968;22:281–393.

41. Andermann A, Blancquaert I, Beauchamp S, Déry V. Revisiting Wilson and Jungner in the genomic age: a review of screening criteria over the past 40 years. Bull World Health Organ. 2008;86:317–9.
42. McKinlay CJD, Chase JG, Dickson J, Harris DL, Alsweiler JM, Harding JE. Continuous glucose monitoring in neonates a review. Matern Health Neonatol Perinatol. 2017;3:18.
43. Tiberi E, Cota F, Barone G, Romano V, Iannotta R, Romagnoli C, Zecca E. Continuous glucose monitoring in preterm infants: evaluation by a modified Clarke error grid. Ital J Pediatr. 2016;42:29.
44. Harris DH, Battin MR, Wesson PJ, Harding JE. Continuous glucose monitoring in newborn babies at risk of hypoglycemia. J Pediatr. 2010;157:198–202 e1.
45. Uettwiller F, Chemin A, Bonnmaison E, Favaris G, Saliba E, Labarthe F. Real time continuous glucose monitoring reduces the episodes of hypoglycemia episodes: a randomized trial in very low birth weight neonates. PLoS One. 2015;10:e0116255.
46. McKinlay CJD, Alsweiler JM, Anstice NS, Burakevych N, Chakraborty A, Chase JG, Gamble GD, Harris DL, Jacobs RJ, Jiang Y, Paudel N, San Diego RJ, Thompson B, Wouldes TA, Harding JE, Children With Hypoglycemia and their Later Development (CHYLD) Study Team. Association of neonatal glycemia with neurodevelopmental outcomes at 45 years. JAMA Pediatr. 2017;171:972–83.
47. Harris DL, Gamble GD, Weston PI, Harding JE. What happens to blood glucose concentrations after oral treatment for neonatal hypoglycemia. J Pediatr. 2017;190:136–41.
48. Flaherman VJ, Gay B, Scott C, Avins A, Lee KA, Newman TB. Randomized trial comparing hand expression with breast pumping for mothers of term newborns feeding poorly. Arch Dis Child Fetal Neonatal Ed. 2012;97:F18–23.
49. Saint L, Smith M, Hartman PE. The yield and nutrient content of colostrum and milk of women from giving birth to 1 month post-partum. Br J Nutr. 1984;52:87–95.
50. Harris DL, Weston PI, Signal M, Chase JG, Harding JE. Dextrose gel for neonatal hypoglycemia (the sugar babies study), a randomized double blind placebo controlled trial. Lancet. 2013;382:2077–83.
51. St Clair SL, Dai DWT, Harris DL, Gamble GD, McKinlay CJD, Nivins S, Shah RK, Thompson B, Harding JE, CHYLD Study Group. Mid-childhood outcomes after dextrose gel treatment of neonatal hypoglycemia: follow up of sugar babies randomized trial. Neonatology. 2023;120:90–102.
52. Lillen LD, Pildes RS, Srinivasan G, Voora S, Yeh TF. Treatment of neonatal hypoglycemia with minibolus and intravenous glucose infusion. J Pediatr. 1980;97:295–8.
53. Rozance PI, Hay WW Jr. New approaches to management of neonatal hypoglycemia. Matern Health Neonatal Perinatol. 2016;2:3.
54. Sen S, Cherkerizian S, Turner D, Monthé-Drèze C, Abdulhayoglu E, Zupancic JAF. A graded approach to intravenous dextrose for neonatal hypoglycemia decreases blood glucose variability, time in the neonatal intensive care unit, and cost of stay. J Pediatr. 2021;231:74–80.

Chapter 7
Prophylactic and Treatment Approaches to Prevent and Treat Neonatal Hypoglycemia

Jane Alsweiler, Kristin Harrison Ginsberg, and Jane Harding

Introduction

Neonatal hypoglycemia is among the most common metabolic abnormalities encountered in newborn infants, and it is also one of the most common reasons for medical intervention in the early postnatal period [1]. Hypoglycemia most often occurs in the first hours and days after birth, as infants transition from a continuous placental glucose supply *in utero* to intermittent enteral (milk) feeding [2]. (See Fig. 7.1).

Neonatal hypoglycemia affects infants across the full spectrum of gestational age and birth weight. The incidence is highest among infants of mothers with diabetes, born preterm, and those who are small or large for gestational age. However, clinically significant hypoglycemia also occurs in infants without recognized risk factors, complicating screening approaches and raising concern about missed or delayed diagnosis [2, 4].

As glucose is the major energy source for the brain, severe neonatal hypoglycemia can be life-threatening and cause brain injury [5]. Prospective cohort studies have found an association between neonatal hypoglycemia with impaired neurodevelopmental outcomes in early childhood [6, 7] and academic performance in mid-childhood [8]. Systematic reviews and a population-based cohort study further support an association between neonatal hypoglycemia and childhood neurodevelopmental outcomes, although findings are variable and may depend on the frequency, duration, and severity of hypoglycemic exposure [9, 10].

J. Alsweiler (✉) · K. H. Ginsberg
Department of Paediatrics: Child and Youth Health, School of Medicine, University of Auckland, Auckland, New Zealand
e-mail: j.alsweiler@auckland.ac.nz

J. Harding
Liggins Institute, University of Auckland, Auckland, New Zealand

D. H. Adamkin, W. W. Hay, Jr. (eds.), *Disorders of Neonatal Glycemia*,
https://doi.org/10.1007/978-3-032-29094-6_7

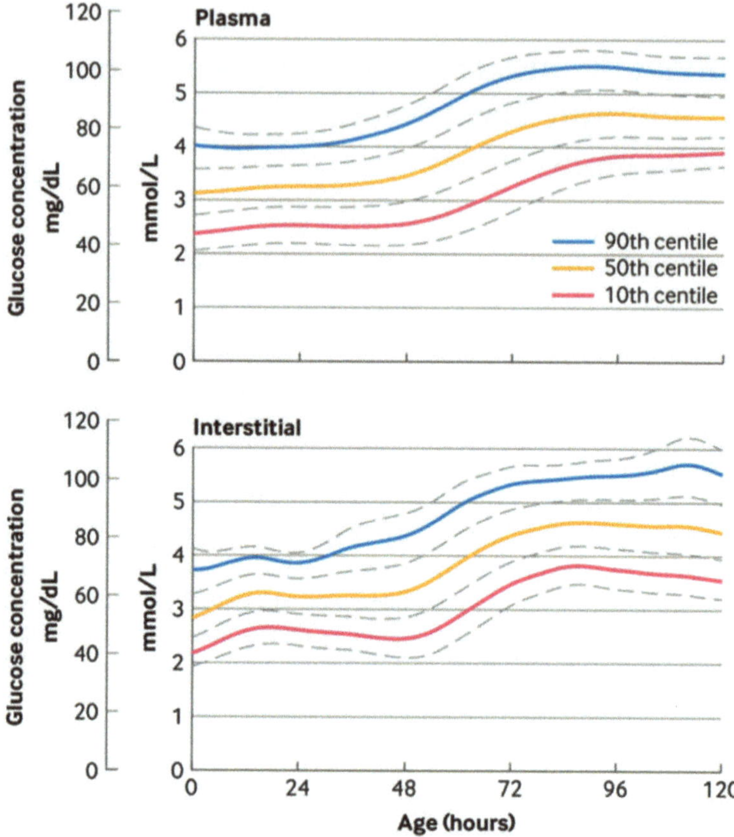

Fig. 7.1 Centiles of plasma and interstitial concentrations of glucose over the first 5 days in healthy term newborns. The 10th centile, in the period from two to 48 h after birth, is about 2.6 mmol/L. (Adapted and reproduced with permission from Harris et al. [3])

Given the potential adverse outcomes of neonatal hypoglycemia (both short- and long-term), prevention strategies that minimize hypoglycemic exposure and treatment approaches that restore and maintain euglycemia are important [1]. However, defining when hypoglycemia is clinically problematic has been challenging, and treatment protocols have historically varied widely [4]. Treatments vary in use dependent on the severity of neonatal hypoglycemia, from feeding strategies and oral dextrose gel to more invasive treatments, with varying effectiveness and side effects [1]. Currently, no prophylactic or treatment strategies have been shown to improve long-term neurodevelopmental outcomes [11].

This chapter reviews current evidence relating to prophylactic and treatment approaches to neonatal hypoglycemia.

Prevention of Neonatal Hypoglycemia

Antenatal and Perinatal Factors

Strategies to reduce the risk of neonatal hypoglycemia before birth have been investigated. The most common risk factor for neonatal hypoglycemia is diabetes in pregnancy. The rates of type 2 diabetes and gestational diabetes, and therefore the incidence of infants requiring screening for neonatal hypoglycemia, have been climbing in part due to the obesity epidemic [12]. Interventions that reduce the incidence of diabetes in pregnancy could be important in reducing the incidence of neonatal hypoglycemia. Lifestyle interventions and myo-inositol in at risk populations are effective at reducing the risk of gestational diabetes [13]. However, most antenatal lifestyle intervention trials did not assess neonatal hypoglycemia, and thus it is unknown whether the reduced incidence of gestational diabetes observed in these trials would reduce neonatal hypoglycemia. In contrast, among women with gestational diabetes, prenatal lifestyle interventions have been found to reduce the risk of neonatal hypoglycemia [14].

Optimising maternal glycemic control in women with pregestational or gestational diabetes reduces fetal exposure to hyperglycemia and may attenuate fetal hyperinsulinism, potentially lowering the risk of postnatal hypoglycemia. However, treatment of women with gestational diabetes, while reducing serious perinatal complications, does not reduce the incidence of neonatal hypoglycemia requiring intravenous dextrose [15]. A systematic review of randomized trials of tighter glycemic targets compared with standard targets for women with gestational diabetes also found no effect of tighter glycemic control on neonatal hypoglycemia [16]. However, a systematic review of tighter compared with less tight glycemic control during the intrapartum period reported very low certainty evidence that this may reduce neonatal hypoglycemia in women with diabetes [17].

While there are antenatal strategies that may reduce the incidence of neonatal hypoglycemia, antenatal interventions can also increase the incidence of neonatal hypoglycemia. Antenatal corticosteroids, given to pregnant women at risk of preterm birth to reduce the incidence of perinatal mortality and other significant complications of prematurity [18], increase the incidence of neonatal hypoglycemia [19]. However, this was not associated with an increase in subsequent neurodevelopmental impairment [20], and recent evidence suggests this effect may be ameliorated by giving metformin to women receiving antenatal corticosteroids [21].

Perinatal practices that support physiological transition may also contribute to prevention. Delayed umbilical cord clamping improves early circulatory stability and iron stores and may support metabolic adaptation, although there is little evidence that it reduces the risk of neonatal hypoglycemia [22]. Immediate postnatal care that minimizes cold stress, avoids unnecessary separation, and supports early mother–infant contact may reduce energy expenditure and facilitate early feeding [10].

Early Feeding

Initiation of feeding soon (within the first hour) after birth provides an exogenous energy source and stimulates endocrine responses that support glucose homeostasis, and may be associated with a reduction in neonatal hypoglycemia [23]. Skin-to-skin contact supports normothermia, reduces stress responses, and facilitates feeding behaviours, and may lead to a large reduction in the incidence of neonatal hypoglycemia as well as other benefits [24].

In some infants, particularly those with limited metabolic reserves or hyperinsulinism, breastfeeding alone may be insufficient to prevent hypoglycemia in the first days after birth. Colostrum volumes are small, and early milk intake may be limited. Supplemental feeding with expressed breast milk, donor milk, or infant formula is therefore commonly used when feeds are delayed or inadequate, although there is limited evidence to support this practice to prevent neonatal hypoglycemia [25]. Overly aggressive supplementation may disrupt breastfeeding establishment and increase parental anxiety [26].

Expression of breast milk before or after birth is frequently recommended for women whose infants are considered at increased risk of hypoglycemia. While antenatal expression appears safe [27], particularly in women with diabetes, evidence that it reduces neonatal hypoglycemia is limited [2, 28]. Expressed breastmilk itself is not associated with a reduction in neonatal hypoglycemia, although breastfeeding may reduce the risk of recurrent neonatal hypoglycemia [16].

Temperature Regulation

Thermal stress substantially increases metabolic demand and glucose utilization in the newborn, so temperature regulation is important. Newborns, particularly those born preterm, small for gestational age, or with limited energy reserves, are vulnerable to hypoglycemia when exposed to hypothermia or even mild cold stress, as cold exposure activates non-shivering thermogenesis, leading to increased oxygen consumption and accelerated depletion of limited hepatic glycogen stores [29]. Maintenance of a neutral thermal environment reduces unnecessary metabolic expenditure and supports glucose homeostasis during the critical postnatal transition.

Clinical strategies to maintain normothermia include immediate drying at birth, use of warm delivery environments, skin-to-skin contact, appropriate clothing and swaddling, and thermal support such as plastic wraps, radiant warmers or incubators for preterm or unwell infants. These measures are emphasized in international neonatal care guidance, which recognizes thermal protection as a foundational component of essential newborn care and a contributor to metabolic stability, including prevention of hypoglycemia [30].

Prophylactic Dextrose Gel

Dextrose gel is non-invasive, inexpensive, and can be administered buccally without separating mother and infant. In large randomized controlled trials of infants at risk of neonatal hypoglycemia, prophylactic dextrose gel given at 1 h of age reduced the incidence of hypoglycemia (defined as blood glucose concentration <2.6 mmol/l (47 mg/dl) [31, 32]. However, prophylactic dextrose gel did not reduce NICU admission, and longitudinal follow-up studies of infants enrolled in prophylactic dextrose gel trials have not demonstrated an improvement in neurodevelopment in early childhood [17, 33] and have raised concerns that there may be adverse effects [34]. In contrast, the use of dextrose gel to treat neonatal hypoglycemia has not raised any concerns about long-term neurodevelopmental outcomes to date [35, 36], although the evidence remains uncertain and more research is required. Importantly, the threshold for acceptable risk differs between prophylactic use and treatment, as prophylaxis exposes infants who may never develop hypoglycemia to potential adverse effects. For these reasons, prophylactic dextrose gel in infants at risk of neonatal hypoglycemia is not recommended for routine use.

Secondary Prevention: Screening

Targeted glucose monitoring is used for the early identification of clinically significant hypoglycemia in infants at risk. Early detection enables timely, low-burden interventions, such as feeding support or administration of oral dextrose gel, which may reduce the risk of prolonged, severe, or recurrent hypoglycemia. Major professional bodies, including the American Academy of Pediatrics, the Pediatric Endocrine Society, and the British Association of Perinatal Medicine, recommend selective (risk-based) screening rather than universal glucose monitoring, focusing on infants with recognized risk factors such as preterm birth, abnormal fetal growth, maternal diabetes, antenatal corticosteroid exposure, or perinatal stress [2, 28, 37]. A large retrospective cohort study conducted over a 14-year-period estimated 25% of babies in one tertiary hospital would meet existing risk-based screening guidelines (Fig. 7.2) [12].

However, screening of infants at risk for neonatal hypoglycemia with blood glucose monitoring does not meet several screening test principles. Specifically, the long-term neurodevelopmental outcomes of transient neonatal hypoglycemia are not well understood and there is no direct evidence from randomized controlled trials that treatment of hypoglycemia improves long-term neurodevelopmental outcomes [38].

Screening guidelines emphasize both timing and thresholds for intervention. At-risk infants are typically screened within the first hours after birth, with continued monitoring during the early transitional period when glucose instability is most likely. Because definitive diagnostic thresholds for hypoglycemia remain uncertain, guidelines use operational thresholds, i.e. values at which intervention is recommended to prevent potential neurological harm rather than to define disease [2, 28]. This approach

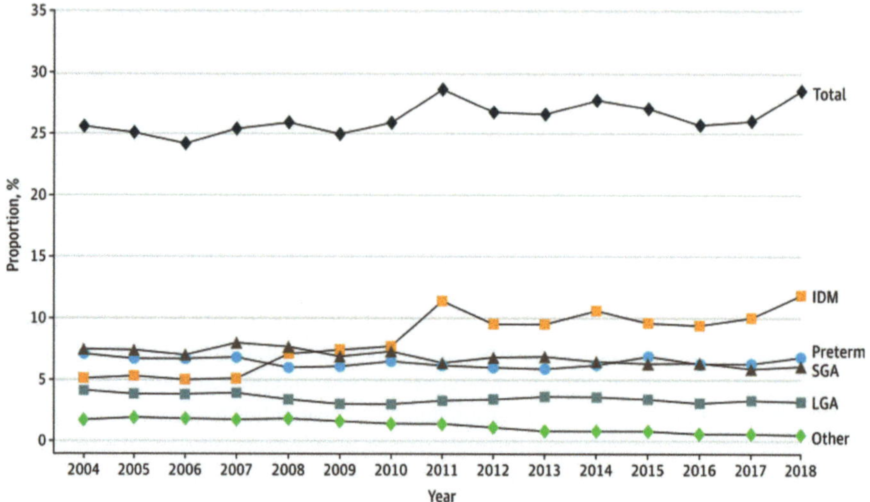

Fig. 7.2 Eligibility of infants born at Auckland City Hospital for neonatal hypoglycemia screening. IDM infants of diabetic mother, SGA small for gestational age, LGA large for gestational age. (Republished with permission from O'Brien et al. [12])

reflects evidence that neonatal hypoglycemia can be asymptomatic yet associated with later adverse neurodevelopmental outcomes [7, 8], while also considering the harms of overdiagnosis, including unnecessary separation of mother and infant, disruption of breastfeeding, and repeated painful blood tests for infants [12].

The utility of screening further depends on measurement accuracy and clinical interpretation. Point-of-care glucose meters are widely used for screening but are less reliable at low glucose concentrations and may be affected by neonatal hematocrit and perfusion, necessitating confirmatory laboratory measurement when results approach treatment thresholds or are discordant with the infant's clinical condition [12].

Studies using continuous glucose monitoring offer promise in measurement improvement and have provided further insight into neonatal glucose patterns. These studies demonstrate that clinically unrecognized hypoglycemia is common, particularly in infants at increased risk, and that intermittent blood sampling may underestimate the duration and frequency of low-glucose exposure [39, 40]. While these observations have improved understanding of neonatal hypoglycemia, continuous glucose monitoring is not currently recommended for routine clinical use in term infants [2, 28].

Conclusion: Prevention

Prevention of neonatal hypoglycemia requires a multifaceted approach that spans antenatal care, perinatal practices, and early feeding support. While transient low glucose concentrations are common during normal adaptation, structured prevention pathways are particularly important for infants at increased risk. Current evidence supports lifestyle interventions to reduce the incidence of gestational diabetes, and practices that promote thermal stability and early feeding. Ongoing refinement of screening strategies and research into operational thresholds is important to balance prevention of harmful hypoglycemia against the risks of overtreatment.

Treatment of Neonatal Hypoglycemia

Feeding as Initial Management

Feeding is usually the first therapeutic response for infants identified with hypoglycemia, particularly those who are clinically well or have mild hypoglycemia. In infants with established hypoglycemia, supplemental feeding with expressed breast milk, donor human milk, or infant formula is frequently used when breastfeeding is delayed or ineffective. Observational cohort studies suggest that formula feeding is associated with modest increases in blood glucose concentrations, whereas expressed breast milk or direct breastfeeding is not effective at increasing blood glucose concentrations [16]. Despite this, breastfeeding has been associated with a reduced risk of recurrent hypoglycemia, possibly mediated by non-nutritional mechanisms such as stimulation of gastrointestinal hormones that influence insulin secretion and glucose utilization [16]. A systematic review of randomized controlled trials found infant formula may be more effective than dextrose gel in correcting hypoglycemia and more effective than breastfeeding in reducing the risk of recurrent hypoglycemia, although the certainty of evidence is low [25].

A pragmatic approach to feeding management therefore involves ongoing support for breastfeeding while recognizing its limitations for acute glucose correction. Adjunctive therapies should be considered when hypoglycemia is detected. Although antenatal or postnatal expression of breast milk is commonly recommended for infants at risk of hypoglycemia, current evidence does not demonstrate a clear effect on neonatal glucose concentrations or hypoglycemia incidence, and this practice should be viewed primarily as a strategy to support feeding rather than as a treatment in its own right [26].

Dextrose Gel

Oral dextrose gel has become a central component of first-line treatment for neonatal hypoglycemia in late preterm and term infants [33]. The gel is typically administered as 0.5 mL/kg of 40% dextrose (200 mg/kg glucose), massaged into the buccal mucosa and followed by a feed. Buccal administration allows rapid absorption while avoiding intravenous access and separation of mother and infant.

Randomized controlled trial evidence demonstrates that dextrose gel is more effective than feeding alone for reversal of hypoglycemia and reduces the risk of treatment failure, intravenous glucose therapy, and admission to neonatal intensive care units [41, 42]. Importantly, use of dextrose gel has been associated with higher rates of breastfeeding at discharge, reflecting its compatibility with family-centered care.

Follow-up studies of infants treated with dextrose gel have not identified adverse effects on neurodevelopment in early or mid-childhood, providing reassurance regarding the safety of early glucose supplementation [6, 41]. Clinical protocols typically limit the number of gel doses administered within a defined period, not because of known toxicity, but to prompt reassessment and escalation of care in infants with persistent hypoglycemia.

Oral Sucrose

Oral sucrose has been used in some settings as an alternative to dextrose for the treatment or prevention of neonatal hypoglycemia, particularly where dextrose gel is unavailable. From a physiological perspective, sucrose is a disaccharide composed of glucose and fructose and must be digested before absorption, potentially delaying or attenuating any increase in blood glucose concentration.

Clinical trials evaluating sucrose administration in newborn infants have reported inconsistent effects on blood glucose concentrations, with some studies demonstrating no benefit compared with feeding alone. Overall, the quality of evidence is low, and sucrose appears less effective than dextrose for rapid correction of hypoglycemia [1]. As a result, sucrose is generally not recommended as a preferred treatment when dextrose gel is available.

Intravenous Dextrose

Intravenous dextrose is indicated for infants with severe, persistent, or symptomatic hypoglycemia, or when enteral interventions fail to restore euglycemia. Initial infusion rates are typically aligned with estimated endogenous glucose production, with subsequent adjustments to infusion rate, glucose concentration, or both to maintain target blood glucose concentrations [2, 28].

The role of an initial intravenous bolus remains controversial. Bolus administration of 1–2 mL/kg of 10% dextrose can rapidly increase blood glucose concentrations; however, concerns have been raised regarding subsequent glycemic instability. Observational data suggest that infants treated with intravenous dextrose are more likely to experience high and unstable glucose concentrations than those treated with enteral approaches, and greater glucose variability following neonatal hypoglycemia has been associated with adverse neurodevelopmental outcomes [7].

In response to these concerns, several guidelines recommend reserving bolus therapy for infants with severe or symptomatic hypoglycemia, while initiating continuous infusion without a bolus in less severe cases [28, 43]. Graded approaches to intravenous glucose administration, including tailoring bolus use and infusion rates to the severity of hypoglycemia, may improve glucose stability and reduce length of neonatal unit stay, although high-quality randomized trial evidence remains limited [1].

Glucagon and Other Pharmacological Treatments

Glucagon may be considered in infants whose hypoglycemia is difficult to stabilize with glucose alone, particularly when inappropriate insulin secretion is suspected. By stimulating hepatic glucose production, glucagon targets a key mechanism underlying hypoglycemia in these infants. It also has the advantage of being able to be given intramuscularly, which can be useful when urgent hypoglycemia treatment is required and intravenous access is difficult. A recent systematic review reported that glucagon administration is associated with short-term increases in blood glucose concentrations, although recurrent hypoglycemia was common and overall certainty of evidence was low [44].

Some infants with hyperinsulinemic hypoglycemia demonstrate inadequate cortisol counter-regulatory responses, suggesting a potential role for corticosteroid supplementation in selected cases [45]. Evidence supporting routine use of glucocorticoids is limited, and such therapy is generally reserved for infants with persistent or refractory hypoglycemia under specialist supervision.

Diazoxide targets the cause of hyperinsulinemia by directly reducing insulin secretion. It has mainly been used in infants with confirmed persistent hyperinsulinemic hypoglycemia rather than as part of routine management for transitional neonatal hypoglycemia [28]. Recent evidence has shown that low dose oral diazoxide may be effective at reducing treatment time and duration of hypoglycemia in infants with severe or recurrent hypoglycemia [46]. However, as diazoxide in infants at higher doses can cause significant adverse events, including pulmonary hypertension and congestive heart failure, further research is required to understand the safety and efficacy of diazoxide in infants with transient hypoglycemia before it can be used routinely.

Conclusion: Treatment

Treatment of neonatal hypoglycemia requires careful balancing of timely correction of low glucose concentrations against the potential harms of intervention. Many infants respond to feeding and oral dextrose gel, while a subset require intravenous therapy or additional pharmacological support. Evidence increasingly supports minimally invasive approaches that restore euglycemia while preserving maternal–infant contact and supporting breastfeeding. Individualised treatment strategies, informed by clinical status, underlying pathophysiology, and response to therapy, remain central to optimising outcomes.

Longer-Term Adverse Outcomes of Neonatal Hypoglycemia

The potential long-term consequences of neonatal hypoglycemia are of particular concern because of the vulnerability of the developing brain in early life. Glucose is the primary energy substrate for the neonatal brain, and cerebral glucose utilization is high relative to body size during the neonatal period [5]. As a result, recurrent, prolonged, or severe hypoglycemia has been associated with an increased risk of neurological injury and adverse neurodevelopmental outcomes [47].

Evidence regarding longer-term outcomes has strengthened substantially over the past decade. Prospective cohort studies have demonstrated associations between neonatal hypoglycemia and adverse neurodevelopmental outcomes in early childhood. In the largest follow-up cohort to date, neonatal hypoglycemia was associated with an increased risk of neurosensory impairment at 2 years of age [6] (Table 7.1).

While, in the Children with Hypoglycemia and Their Later Development (CHYLD) study, neonatal hypoglycemia was not associated with an increased risk of neurosensory impairment at 2 years of age [39]. However, follow-up of the CHYLD cohort at 4.5 years identified associations between neonatal hypoglycemia and low executive function and visual–motor integration, suggesting that some effects of early hypoglycemia may not be fully apparent until later childhood [7].

Longer-term follow-up into mid-childhood has extended these findings further. Neonatal hypoglycemia has been associated with differences in academic achievement, including performance in literacy and numeracy, indicating that early disturbances in glucose homeostasis may have implications for later educational outcomes [8, 48]. However, outcomes are heterogeneous, and many infants exposed to neonatal hypoglycemia do not experience measurable impairment.

Systematic reviews and population-based studies suggest that the risk of adverse outcomes following neonatal hypoglycemia is influenced by the burden of hypoglycemic exposure, including the frequency, duration, and severity of low glucose concentrations, as well as the presence of coexisting risk factors [9, 10]. These findings support a focus on minimising cumulative hypoglycemic exposure rather than reliance on a single glucose threshold.

Neuroimaging studies offer additional biological plausibility for these neurodevelopmental findings. Magnetic resonance imaging performed in mid-childhood has identified associations between neonatal hypoglycemia and differences in brain structure, including altered brain volumes and white matter microstructure [49]. The clinical significance of these findings remains an area of ongoing investigation.

Follow-up studies of infants treated with oral dextrose gel, either therapeutically or prophylactically, have not demonstrated adverse neurodevelopmental outcomes in early or mid-childhood; however, they have also not demonstrated benefits over placebo [34, 35, 41, 50, 51].

Table 7.1 Associations between neonatal hypoglycemia and neurosensory impairment at corrected age 2 years[a]

Primary outcome	No./total no. (%)	RD/MD (95% CI)	RR (95% CI)	Adjusted RR/MD (95% CI)[b]	*P* value
Normoglycemia	125/704 (17.8)				
Hypoglycemia[c]	111/487 (22.8)	5.04 (0.36 to 9.72)	1.28 (1.02 to 1.61)	1.28 (1.01 to 1.60)	0.04
Severity of hypoglycemia[d,e]					0.02
Mild	81/381 (21.3)	3.50 (−1.49 to 8.49)	1.20 (0.93 to 1.54)	1.18 (0.92 to 1.52)	0.19
Severe	30/106 (28.3)	10.55 (1.51 to 19.59)	1.59 (1.13 to 2.25)	1.68 (1.20 to 2.36)	0.003

[a]*MD* mean difference, *RD* risk difference, *RR* risk ratio
[b]Defined as any of the following: blindness (visual acuity <3/60 or >1.3 logMAR), hearing impairment requiring aids, cerebral palsy, developmental delay (Bayley-III cognitive, language, or motor composite score <85), or performance-based executive function total score more than 1.5 SD below the cohort mean
[c]Adjusted for study site, primary reason for risk of hypoglycemia, socioeconomic decile at birth, and multiple births
[d]An episode of hypoglycemia was defined as 1 or more episode of consecutive blood glucose concentrations less than 47 mg/dL (to convert glucose to millimoles per liter, multiply by 0.0555)
[e]The severity of hypoglycemia was defined as none (all blood glucose concentrations ≥47 mg/dL), mild (≥1 episode of ≥36 and <47 mg/dL), and severe (≥1 episode of <36 mg/dL)
Republished with permission from Edwards et al. [6]

Conclusion: Longer-Term Adverse Outcomes

Neonatal hypoglycemia is associated with an increased risk of adverse neurodevelopmental and academic outcomes, particularly when exposure is recurrent, prolonged, and severe. Evidence from prospective cohort studies, systematic reviews, and neuroimaging supports efforts to minimize hypoglycemic burden while avoiding unnecessary intervention. Further research is needed to refine risk stratification and follow-up practices for infants at greatest risk.

References

1. Harding JE, Alsweiler JM, Edwards TE, McKinlay CJ. Neonatal hypoglycaemia. BMJ Med. 2024;3(1):e000544. https://doi.org/10.1136/bmjmed-2023-000544.
2. Adamkin DH, Committee on Fetus and Newborn. Postnatal glucose homeostasis in late-preterm and term infants. Pediatrics. 2011;127(3):e20103851. https://doi.org/10.1542/peds.2010-3851.
3. Harris DL, Weston PJ, Gamble GD, Harding JE. Glucose profiles in healthy term infants in the first 5 days: the glucose in well babies (GLOW) study. J Pediatr. 2020;223:34–41.e4. https://doi.org/10.1016/j.jpeds.2020.02.079.

4. Cornblath M, Hawdon JM, Williams AF, et al. Controversies regarding definition of neonatal hypoglycemia: suggested operational thresholds. Pediatrics. 2000;105(5):1141–5. https://doi.org/10.1542/peds.105.5.1141.
5. De Angelis LC, Brigati G, Polleri G, et al. Neonatal hypoglycemia and brain vulnerability. Front Endocrinol. 2021;12:634305. https://doi.org/10.3389/fendo.2021.634305.
6. Edwards T, Alsweiler JM, Gamble GD, et al. Neurocognitive outcomes at age 2 years after neonatal hypoglycemia in a cohort of participants from the hPOD randomized trial. JAMA Netw Open. 2022;5(10):e2235989. https://doi.org/10.1001/jamanetworkopen.2022.35989.
7. McKinlay CJD, Alsweiler JM, Anstice NS, et al. Association of neonatal glycemia with neurodevelopmental outcomes at 4.5 years. JAMA Pediatr. 2017;171(10):972. https://doi.org/10.1001/jamapediatrics.2017.1579.
8. Shah R, Dai DWT, Alsweiler JM, et al. Association of neonatal hypoglycemia with academic performance in mid-childhood. JAMA. 2022;327(12):1158. https://doi.org/10.1001/jama.2022.0992.
9. Wickström R, Skiöld B, Petersson G, Stephansson O, Altman M. Moderate neonatal hypoglycemia and adverse neurological development at 2–6 years of age. Eur J Epidemiol. 2018;33(10):1011–20. https://doi.org/10.1007/s10654-018-0425-5.
10. Boluyt N, Van Kempen A, Offringa M. Neurodevelopment after neonatal hypoglycemia: a systematic review and design of an optimal future study. Pediatrics. 2006;117(6):2231–43. https://doi.org/10.1542/peds.2005-1919.
11. Alsweiler JM, Harris DL, Harding JE, McKinlay CJD. Strategies to improve neurodevelopmental outcomes in babies at risk of neonatal hypoglycaemia. Lancet Child Adolesc Health. 2021;5(7):513–23. https://doi.org/10.1016/S2352-4642(20)30387-4.
12. O'Brien M, Gilchrist C, Sadler L, Hegarty JE, Alsweiler JM. Infants eligible for neonatal hypoglycemia screening: a systematic review. JAMA Pediatr. 2023;177(11):1187. https://doi.org/10.1001/jamapediatrics.2023.3957.
13. Takele WW, Vesco KK, Josefson J, et al. Effective interventions in preventing gestational diabetes mellitus: a systematic review and meta-analysis. Commun Med. 2024;4(1):75. https://doi.org/10.1038/s43856-024-00491-1.
14. Wang YH, Zhou HH, Nie Z, et al. Lifestyle intervention during pregnancy in patients with gestational diabetes mellitus and the risk of neonatal hypoglycemia: a systematic review and meta-analysis. Front Nutr. 2022;9:962151. https://doi.org/10.3389/fnut.2022.962151.
15. Crowther CA, Hiller JE, Moss JR, McPhee AJ, Jeffries WS, Robinson JS. Effect of treatment of gestational diabetes mellitus on pregnancy outcomes. N Engl J Med. 2005;352(24):2477–86. https://doi.org/10.1056/NEJMoa042973.
16. Harris DL, Gamble GD, Weston PJ, Harding JE. What happens to blood glucose concentrations after oral treatment for neonatal hypoglycemia? J Pediatr. 2017;190:136–41. https://doi.org/10.1016/j.jpeds.2017.06.034.
17. Ulyatt CM, Roberts LF, Crowther CA, Harding JE, Lin L. Intrapartum maternal glycaemic control for the prevention of neonatal hypoglycaemia: a systematic review and meta-analysis. BMC Pregnancy Childbirth. 2024;24(1):423. https://doi.org/10.1186/s12884-024-06615-8.
18. McGoldrick E, Stewart F, Parker R, Dalziel SR. Antenatal corticosteroids for accelerating fetal lung maturation for women at risk of preterm birth. Cochrane Database Syst Rev. 2020;2021(2). https://doi.org/10.1002/14651858.CD004454.pub4.
19. Gyamfi-Bannerman C, Thom EA, Blackwell SC, et al. Antenatal betamethasone for women at risk for late preterm delivery. N Engl J Med. 2016;374(14):1311–20. https://doi.org/10.1056/NEJMoa1516783.
20. Gyamfi-Bannerman C, Clifton RG, Tita ATN, et al. Neurodevelopmental outcomes after late preterm antenatal corticosteroids: the ALPS follow-up study. JAMA. 2024;331(19):1629. https://doi.org/10.1001/jama.2024.4303.
21. Yefet E, Massalha M, Talmon G, et al. Metformin, maternal glycemic control, and neonatal hypoglycemia after antenatal steroids: a randomized clinical trial. JAMA Netw Open. 2026;9(1):e2552807. https://doi.org/10.1001/jamanetworkopen.2025.52807.

22. Watson ED, Roberts LF, Harding JE, Crowther CA, Lin L. Umbilical cord milking and delayed cord clamping for the prevention of neonatal hypoglycaemia: a systematic review and meta-analysis. BMC Pregnancy Childbirth. 2024;24(1):248. https://doi.org/10.1186/s12884-024-06427-w.
23. Roberts LF, Harding JE, Crowther CA, Watson E, Wang Z, Lin L. Early feeding for the prevention of neonatal hypoglycaemia: a systematic review and meta-analysis. Neonatology. 2024;121(2):141–56. https://doi.org/10.1159/000535503.
24. Lord LG, Harding JE, Crowther CA, Lin L. Skin-to-skin contact for the prevention of neonatal hypoglycaemia: a systematic review and meta-analysis. BMC Pregnancy Childbirth. 2023;23(1):744. https://doi.org/10.1186/s12884-023-06057-8.
25. Iqbal A, Harding JE, Lin L. Infant formula for the prevention and treatment of neonatal hypoglycaemia: a systematic review and meta-analysis. Acta Paediatr. 2026;115(1):32–42. https://doi.org/10.1111/apa.70325.
26. Oladimeji OI, Harding JE, Crowther CA, Lin L. Expressed breast milk and maternal expression of breast milk for the prevention and treatment of neonatal hypoglycemia: a systematic review and meta-analysis. Matern Health Neonatol Perinatol. 2023;9(1):12. https://doi.org/10.1186/s40748-023-00166-0.
27. Forster DA, Moorhead AM, Jacobs SE, et al. Advising women with diabetes in pregnancy to express breastmilk in late pregnancy (Diabetes and Antenatal Milk Expressing [DAME]): a multicentre, unblinded, randomised controlled trial. Lancet. 2017;389(10085):2204–13. https://doi.org/10.1016/S0140-6736(17)31373-9.
28. Thornton PS, Stanley CA, De Leon DD, et al. Recommendations from the pediatric endocrine society for evaluation and management of persistent hypoglycemia in neonates, infants, and children. J Pediatr. 2015;167(2):238–45. https://doi.org/10.1016/j.jpeds.2015.03.057.
29. Kurz C, Roeper M, Welters A, et al. Relationship of neonatal hypothermia and hypoglycemia in late preterm and term born neonates. Mol Cell Pediatr. 2025;12(1):15. https://doi.org/10.1186/s40348-025-00204-1.
30. Liu J, Wu S, Zhu X. Advances in the prevention and treatment of neonatal hypothermia in early birth. Ther Hypothermia Temp Manag. 2022;12(2):51–6. https://doi.org/10.1089/ther.2021.0036.
31. Harding JE, Hegarty JE, Crowther CA, et al. Evaluation of oral dextrose gel for prevention of neonatal hypoglycemia (hPOD): a multicenter, double-blind randomized controlled trial. PLoS Med. 2021;18(1):e1003411. https://doi.org/10.1371/journal.pmed.1003411.
32. Hegarty JE, Harding JE, Gamble GD, Crowther CA, Edlin R, Alsweiler JM. Prophylactic oral dextrose gel for newborn babies at risk of neonatal hypoglycaemia: a randomised controlled dose-finding trial (the Pre-hPOD Study). PLoS Med. 2016;13(10):e1002155. https://doi.org/10.1371/journal.pmed.1002155.
33. Roberts L, Lin L, Alsweiler J, Edwards T, Liu G, Harding JE. Oral dextrose gel to prevent hypoglycaemia in at-risk neonates. Cochrane Database Syst Rev. 2023;2023(11). https://doi.org/10.1002/14651858.CD012152.pub4.
34. Edwards T, Alsweiler JM, Crowther CA, et al. Prophylactic oral dextrose gel and neurosensory impairment at 2-year follow-up of participants in the hPOD randomized trial. JAMA. 2022;327(12):1149. https://doi.org/10.1001/jama.2022.2363.
35. Harris DL, Alsweiler JM, Ansell JM, et al. Outcome at 2 years after dextrose gel treatment for neonatal hypoglycemia: follow-up of a randomized trial. J Pediatr. 2016;170:54–59.e2. https://doi.org/10.1016/j.jpeds.2015.10.066.
36. Edwards T, Liu G, Battin M, et al. Oral dextrose gel for the treatment of hypoglycaemia in newborn infants. Cochrane Database Syst Rev. 2022;2022(3). https://doi.org/10.1002/14651858.CD011027.pub3.
37. Levene I, Wilkinson D. Identification and management of neonatal hypoglycaemia in the full-term infant (British Association of Perinatal Medicine—Framework for practice). Arch Dis Child Educ Pract Ed. 2019;104(1):29–32. https://doi.org/10.1136/archdischild-2017-314050.

38. Alsweiler JM, Heather N, Harris DL, McKinlay CJD. Application of the screening test principles to screening for neonatal hypoglycemia. Front Pediatr. 2022;10:1048897. https://doi.org/10.3389/fped.2022.1048897.
39. McKinlay CJD, Alsweiler JM, Ansell JM, et al. Neonatal glycemia and neurodevelopmental outcomes at 2 years. N Engl J Med. 2015;373(16):1507–18. https://doi.org/10.1056/NEJMoa1504909.
40. Harris DL, Battin MR, Weston PJ, Harding JE. Continuous glucose monitoring in newborn babies at risk of hypoglycemia. J Pediatr. 2010;157(2):198–202.e1. https://doi.org/10.1016/j.jpeds.2010.02.003.
41. Griffith R, Hegarty JE, Alsweiler JM, et al. Two-year outcomes after dextrose gel prophylaxis for neonatal hypoglycaemia. Arch Dis Child Fetal Neonatal Ed. 2021;106(3):278–85. https://doi.org/10.1136/archdischild-2020-320305.
42. Harris DL, Weston PJ, Signal M, Chase JG, Harding JE. Dextrose gel for neonatal hypoglycaemia (the sugar babies study): a randomised, double-blind, placebo-controlled trial. Lancet. 2013;382(9910):2077–83. https://doi.org/10.1016/S0140-6736(13)61645-1.
43. Te Tohu Waihonga Guideline Group. Te Tohu Waihonga-Aotearoa New Zealand clinical practice guideline for neonatal hypoglycaemia. Liggins Institute; 2025.
44. Walsh EPG, Alsweiler JM, Ardern J, Hanning SM, Harding JE, McKinlay CJD. Glucagon for neonatal hypoglycaemia: systematic review and meta-analysis. Neonatology. 2022;119(3):285–94. https://doi.org/10.1159/000522415.
45. Hussain K, Hindmarsh P, Aynsley-Green A. Neonates with symptomatic hyperinsulinemic hypoglycemia generate inappropriately low serum cortisol counterregulatory hormonal responses. J Clin Endocrinol Metabol. 2003;88(9):4342–7. https://doi.org/10.1210/jc.2003-030135.
46. Laing D, Walsh EPG, Alsweiler JM, et al. Diazoxide for severe or recurrent neonatal hypoglycemia: a randomized clinical trial. JAMA Netw Open. 2024;7(6):e2415764. https://doi.org/10.1001/jamanetworkopen.2024.15764.
47. Diggikar S, Trif P, Mudura D, et al. Neonatal hypoglycemia and neurodevelopmental outcomes—an updated systematic review and meta-analysis. Life. 2024;14(12):1618. https://doi.org/10.3390/life14121618.
48. Dai DWT, Franke N, McKinlay CJD, et al. Executive function and behaviour problems in school-age children born at risk of neonatal hypoglycaemia. Develop Med Child Neuro. 2023;65(9):1226–37. https://doi.org/10.1111/dmcn.15520.
49. Nivins S, Kennedy E, Thompson B, et al. Associations between neonatal hypoglycaemia and brain volumes, cortical thickness and white matter microstructure in mid-childhood: an MRI study. NeuroImage Clin. 2022;33:102943. https://doi.org/10.1016/j.nicl.2022.102943.
50. Harris DL, Gamble GD, Harding JE. Outcome at 4.5 years after dextrose gel treatment of hypoglycaemia: follow-up of the sugar babies randomised trial. Arch Dis Child Fetal Neonatal Ed. 2023;108(2):121–8. https://doi.org/10.1136/archdischild-2022-324148.
51. St Clair SL, Dai DWT, Harris DL, et al. Mid-childhood outcomes after dextrose gel treatment of neonatal hypoglycaemia: follow-up of the sugar babies randomized trial. Neonatology. 2023;120(1):90–101. https://doi.org/10.1159/000527715.

Part IV
Neonatal Hyperglycemia

Chapter 8
Conditions in the Fetus that Promote Neonatal Hyperglycemia

William W. Hay, Jr.

Neonatal hyperglycemia begins in the fetus. During pregnancy in normal women with normal glucose metabolism, maternal glucose production (GPR) tends to increase in response to increasing glucose utilization by the conceptus (pregnant uterus, placenta and fetus), but maternal GPR does not quite keep up with the increasing transfer of glucose to the conceptus. As a result, maternal and thus fetal plasma glucose concentrations tend to decrease over the second half of gestation (Fig. 8.1) [1].

Maternal insulin resistance in maternal skeletal muscle and adipose tissue tends to develop in late gestation, which helps maintain maternal plasma glucose concentration to support glucose transfer from the maternal plasma to the conceptus.

In normal pregnant women, acute maternal plasma hyperglycemia such as in response to a mid-gestation glucose tolerance test, either with an enteral load of dextrose or glucose-containing beverage or with an intravenous bolus of dextrose (glucose), glucose is transferred to the conceptus and increases fetal plasma glucose concentration. Fetal insulin production, secretion, and plasma concentrations increase in direct response to the acute fetal hyperglycemia. This is commonly seen in fetuses of unstable diabetic mothers, whose glucose concentrations, particularly in response to a high sugar or low complex, simple carbohydrate meal, can increase suddenly and rapidly. Insulin secretion in the fetus begins in the early second trimester and increases in response to glucose stimulation as gestation proceeds.

In pregnant women with type 1, largely insulin dependent diabetes mellitus, hyperglycemia is present from conception throughout gestation, adversely affecting embryonic and fetal development. In pregnant women with gestational diabetes and closely linked obesity and overweight, who now are in pandemic proportions, there is much greater insulin resistance than occurs in normal pregnancies that reduces

W. W. Hay, Jr. (✉)
University of Colorado, Denver, CO, USA
e-mail: bill.hay@ucdenver.edu

D. H. Adamkin, W. W. Hay, Jr. (eds.), *Disorders of Neonatal Glycemia*,
https://doi.org/10.1007/978-3-032-29094-6_8

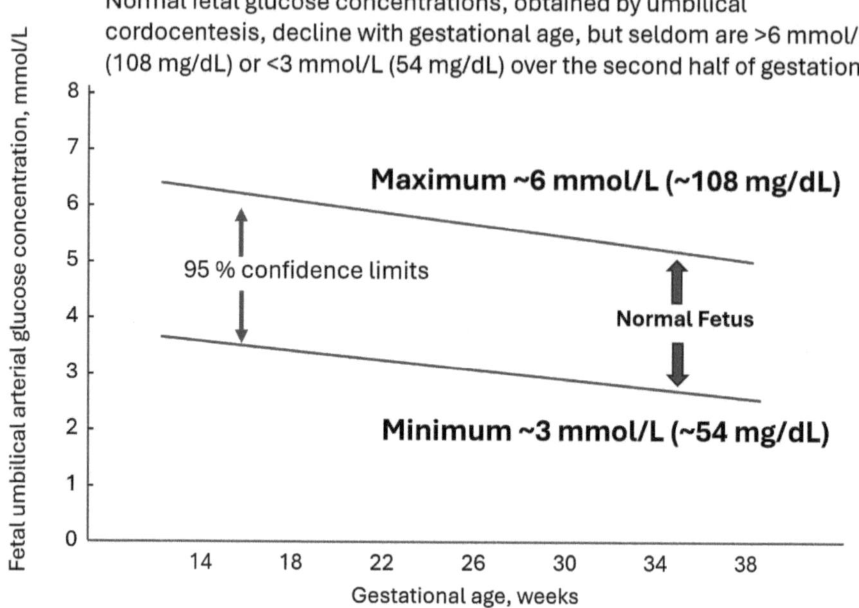

Fig. 8.1 Normal fetal glucose concentrations range between 3.0 mmol/L (54 mg/dL) and 6 mmol/L (108 mg/dL). (Adapted from: Marconi et al. [1])

glucose disposal and promotes chronic maternal and thus fetal hyperglycemia [2]. Gestational diabetes, which is closely linked with obesity and overweight, is increasing among all racial and ethnic groups [3]. Pregnant women with gestational diabetes, obesity, and overweight have increased up to +36% among all racial and ethnic groups over the past 25 years, a significant trend that is greatest in non-Hispanic Asian/Pacific Islanders at +46%. Among the non-Hispanic Asian group, the average annual percentage change (AAPC) in GD rates per 1000 live births significantly ($P < .05$) increased in Asian Indian (2.6%; 95% CI, 2.0%–3.2%), Chinese (6.8%; 95% CI, 4.6%–9.1%), Filipina (4.1%; 95% CI, 1.7%–6.6%), Japanese (4.8%; 95% CI, 1.4%–8.6%), Korean (2.7%; 95% CI, 0.9%–4.7%), and Vietnamese (4.0%; 95% CI, 2.2%–5.9%) ethnicities. Among the Hispanic group, the AAPC in GD rates per 1000 live births significantly increased in Central and South American (3.2%; 95% CI, 0.8%–5.8%), Cuban (3.7%; 95% CI, 1.0%–5.9%), Mexican (3.8%; 95% CI, 2.9%–4.8%), and Puerto Rican (3.4%; 95% CI, 2.4%–4.4%) ethnicities [4]. In the US in the state of Florida, representative of many of the southern and southeastern US states, gestational obesity and overweight, along with gestational diabetes or diabetic-like conditions, is more common among Native Americans and Blacks, while all racial groups have some form of obesity and overweight, from 20% to 40% [5].

GDM women are more susceptible to insulin resistance, which results in maternal hyperglycemia and hyperinsulinemia. Gestational diabetes mellitus (GDM), characterized by gestational hyperglycemia due to insufficient insulin response, poses significant risks to both maternal and offspring health. Pregnant women without diagnosed GDM but mildly hyperglycemic also produce adverse pregnancy outcomes, indicating strong, continuous associations of maternal glucose concentrations below those that are diagnostic of diabetes (pre-gestational or GDM) with increased birth weight and increased cord-blood serum C-peptide in the offspring [6]. Fetal exposure to maternal hyperglycemia leads to short-term complications such as macrosomia and neonatal hypoglycemia and long-term risks including obesity, metabolic syndrome, cardiovascular dysfunction, and type 2 diabetes. The Developmental Origins of Health and Disease (DOHaD) theory explains how maternal hyperglycemia alters fetal programming, increasing susceptibility to the noted metabolic disorders later in life [7]. Mechanisms include epigenetic modifications in genes affecting neuroendocrine activities and metabolism, increasing the risk of obesity and type 2 diabetes in offspring [8].

Fetal Metabolic Adaptations to Gestational Hyperglycemia

How does the fetus adapt metabolically to chronic glucose excess and hyperglycemia? Regardless of how these conditions occur, the fetus gradually develops increased insulin resistance and glucose intolerance. These changes appear to occur in all glucose and insulin-sensitive organs. In fetal sheep exposed to chronic hyperglycemia, Glut 1 and Glut 4 are reduced with sustained hyperglycemia [9], whether induced by chronic dextrose infusions into the maternal circulation or by blocking insulin secretion in the fetus with streptozotocin, a drug that damages pancreatic islet β-cells, or glucagon that enhances pancreatic glucose production (Fig. 8.2) [9–11].

Glucose utilization is decreased under such chronic hyperglycemic conditions at both low (normal) and high insulin concentrations, demonstrating both insulin resistance and reduced glucose utilization rate in response to sustained, marked hyperglycemia (GUR). Chronic hyperglycemia, as studied in fetal sheep in late gestation, also gradually reduces basal and glucose-stimulated insulin secretion. This will gradually add to hyperglycemia induced by the maternal hyperglycemia-induced fetal hyperglycemia (Fig. 8.3) [12].

In human pregnancies, however, this chronic, sustained and marked hyperglycemia is usually confined to long standing and poorly controlled insulin-dependent diabetic women. More commonly, particularly in gestational diabetics (including women with obesity and mild to moderate diabetic-like conditions), pulsatile, meal- and snack-associated hyperglycemia occurs, which produces different insulin secretion patterns (Fig. 8.4) [13, 14].

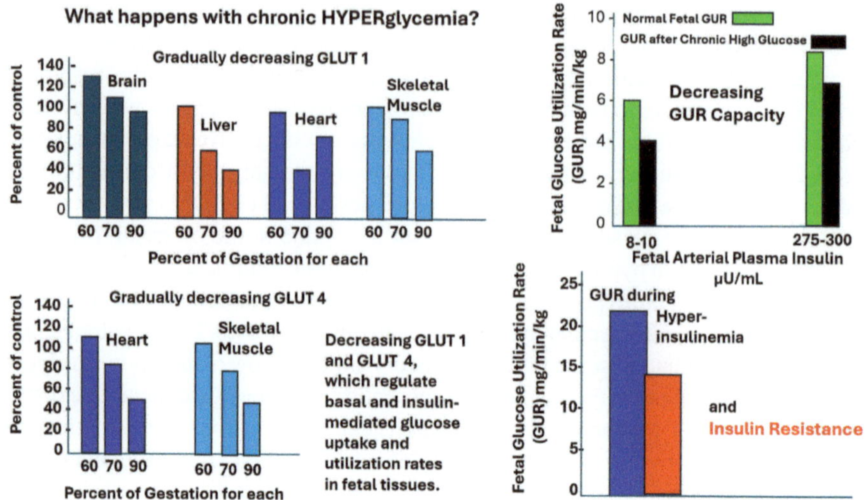

Fig. 8.2 Glucose transporter and glucose metabolic responses to chronic fetal hyperglycemia. (Adapted from: Das et al. [9], Hay Jr. and Meznarich [10], and Hay Jr. et al. [11])

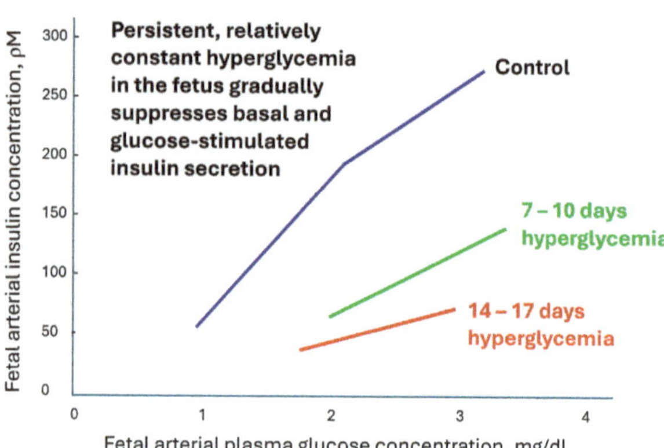

Fig. 8.3 Fetal metabolic adaptations to chronic hyperglycemia. (Adapted from: Carver et al. [12])

When studied in a controlled animal model, the pregnant sheep, fetal glucose-stimulated insulin secretion (GSIS) is most augmented by pulsatile hyperglycemia that is characteristic of gestational diabetics and milder but poorly controlled insulin dependent diabetics [15]. Hypoglycemia suppresses GSIS, but chronic, marked hyperglycemia has the greatest suppression of GSIS. Thus, the magnitude, duration, and pattern of fetal glycemia, directly regulated by maternal plasma glucose concentration, regulates fetal pancreatic insulin secretion capacity (Fig. 8.5) [16].

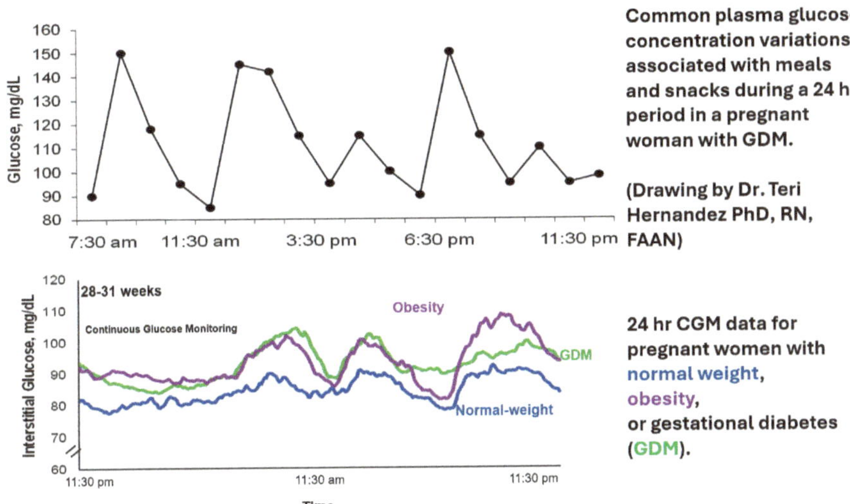

Fig. 8.4 24 h maternal glucose concentration variations in response to intermittent food intake and fasting. (Top Panel Figure drawn by Dr. Teri Hernandez, University of Colorado School of Nursing. Adapted from data in: Hernandez et al. [13, 14])

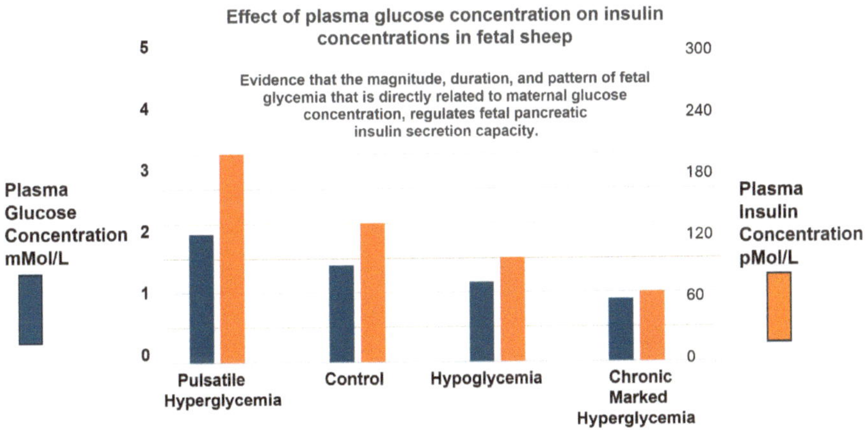

Fig. 8.5 Pulsatile hyperglycemia induces the greatest increase in insulin secretion in contrast to constant, marked hyperglycemia that suppresses insulin secretion. (Adapted from: Carver et al. [16])

IUGR and Effects of Gestational Hyperglycemia, Particularly Fetal Glucose Production

Hyperglycemia is especially a problem in IUGR fetuses due to reduced fetal pancreas development and decreased fetal GSIS (Fig. 8.6) [17].

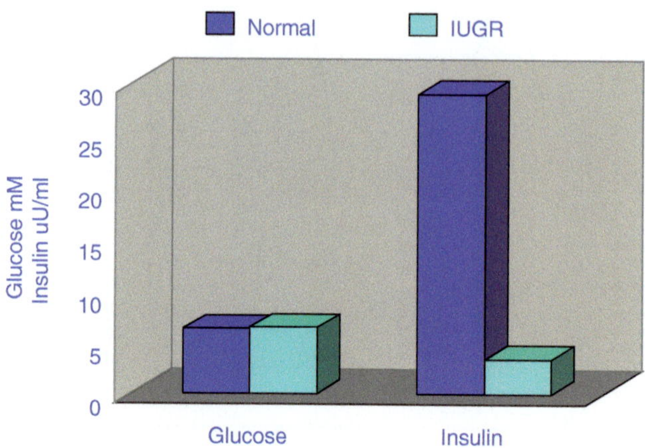

Fig. 8.6 Glucose stimulated insulin secretion is suppressed in IUGR human fetuses. (Adapted from: Nicolini et al. [17])

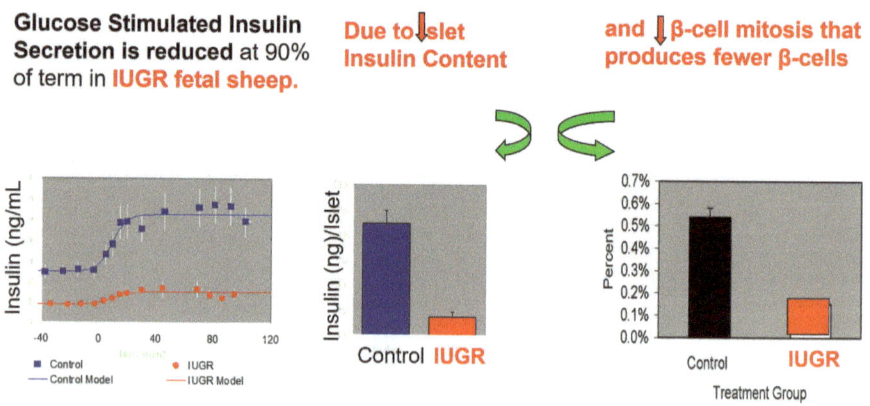

Fig. 8.7 Glucose stimulated insulin secretion is reduced in response to suppression of pancreatic insulin content caused by diminished pancreatic beta-cell mitosis. (Adapted from: Limesand et al. [19])

Insulin secretion from pancreatic B-cells is impaired in all forms of hyperglycemia, especially when chronic. In such conditions, hyperglycemia results in marked glycogen accumulation in the pancreas and increased apoptosis in B-cells. Sulfonylureas have long been known to reverse this suppression of insulin secretion, dissipating glycogen stores, increasing autophagy, restoring B-cell metabolism, and promoting insulin secretion. Insulin has the same effect but acts more slowly [18].

As studied in normal and IUGR fetal sheep, suppressed GSIS occurs because of reduced fetal pancreatic islet insulin content and decreased islet β-cell mitosis that produces fewer β-cells (Fig. 8.7) [19].

The mechanism for these conditions is suppression of GSIS by catecholamines that are increased in IUGR fetuses from placental insufficiency-induced fetal hypoxia [20]. Blocking production and thus plasma concentrations of catecholamines (adrenergic stimulation) increases GSIS, proof that catecholamines are responsible for suppressing GSIS in IUGR fetuses with hypoxia [20, 21]. IUGR fetuses with placental insufficiency, hypoxia, and acidemia also increase glucagon secretion. Glucagon specifically can increase glucose production leading to or augmenting already present glucose concentrations [22, 23].

Counter-hormone production, vasoactive medications (e.g., epinephrine and norepinephrine), or glucocorticoids remain common factors for hyperglycemia. Cortisol (endogenous or exogenous) increases glucose production by activating phosphoenol pyruvate carboxy-kinase and plasma concentrations by activating glycogen phosphorylase that breaks down glycogen to glucose-6-phosphate and glucose-6-phosphatase that is responsible for releasing glucose from hepatocytes into the circulation. Cortisol also increases protein catabolism, increasing plasma concentrations of selected amino acids such as alanine and glutamine that are used for gluconeogenesis. Alanine, arginine, proline, glycine, and lysine stimulate glucagon secretion that in turn enhances gluconeogenesis [24–26]. Commonly used lipid infusions and their products such as free fatty acids (FFA) compete with glucose and decrease its oxidation at the cellular level, while both glycerol and FFA can directly activate gluconeogenesis by induction of several enzymatic pathways. Increased exposure to hyperglycemia is commonly observed in the presence of higher lipids intake ($p = 0.031$) [27]. Birthweight is the strongest predictor of neonatal glucose profile with an inverse relationship between the time spent in hyperglycemia and birthweight ($p = 0.007$), indicating that hyperglycemia itself does not necessarily promote growth or even fat mass gain.

Glycerol also can serve as a fuel for gluconeogenesis. In addition, preterm newborns exhibit a paradoxical response to glucose infusions and glucose levels. Physiologically, infusion of dextrose ≥6 mg/kg/min can suppress hepatic glucose production in children and adults, but the threshold for glucose infusion to suppress glucose production in preterm newborns can be as high as 16 mg/kg/min and plasma glucose concentrations as high as ≥250 mg/dL (13.9 mmol/L). Gluconeogenesis also persists in preterm newborns on parenteral nutrition. Persistent glucose production, despite glucose infusion and hyperglycemia, has been shown in preterm infants even at 2–5 weeks postnatal age [28–33].

Importantly, adrenergic inhibition that results in a greater GSIS responsiveness even though β-cell mass is reduced (by up to 50%–60%) and the maximal stimulatory insulin response tends to be higher. Persistent catecholamine (adrenergic/norepinephrine) suppression of GSIS may be partially explained by higher mRNA concentrations of adrenergic receptors alpha(1D), alpha(2A), and alpha(2B) [34]. Catecholamine (norepinephrine) suppression of GSIS is maintained, in part, by upregulating adrenergic receptor expression, but the beta-cells also appeared to compensate with enhanced GSIS. These observations, while in an animal model, might help to explain how IUGR human infants have a greater propensity for increased GSIS, acute hypoglycemia, and glucose requirements when early postnatal catecholamines decrease after birth. Further contributing to hyperglycemia in IUGR fetuses, also as shown in IUGR fetal sheep, is increased hepatic glucose production due to hepatic insulin resistance that can persist in the neonate [35]. Infusion of insulin does not reduce hepatic glucose production or PCK1 mRNA or PEPCK protein in the IUGR fetus [36, 37].

Fetal Effects of Hyperglycemia in Gestational Diabetes

In addition to IUGR conditions that produce sustained, but variable hyperglycemia, there are many complications of chronic fetal hyperglycemia that are commonly seen in fetuses of diabetic mothers (IDMs) (Table 8.1).

There are many examples of maternal gestational diabetes with hyperglycemia that produce newborn infants with abnormal metabolism. At least one mechanism could be that such mothers have increased oxidative stress during pregnancy. Either in the fetus from hyperglycemia or transferred from the mothers, oxidate stress parameters, sch malondialdehyde (MDA), total antioxidant capacity (TAC), and DNA damage (comet assay, for example) have been increased in neonates born to gestational diabetic mothers [38]. Hyperglycemia also has been shown to inhibit retinoic acid-induced activation of Rac1, prevents differentiation of cortical neurons, and causes oxidative stress in a rat model of diabetic pregnancy [39]. Oxidative stress could produce abnormal cellular development in multiple organs in neonates. Maternal obesity with increased body mass index due to excess body fat mass, generally associated with at least intermittent if not constant maternal hyperglycemia, might lead to oxidative stress in the fetus that produces fetal insulin resistance. One study, in fact, showed that such insulin resistance was positively associated with increased glucose and oxygen uptake by the fetus, which could be responsible for increased fetal growth, particularly of adipose tissue [40].

Table 8.1 Pathological conditions in hyperglycemic IDMs

↑ Fat deposition more than lean mass
↑ Inflammatory fatty infiltration of heart and liver
↑ Cardiac septal hypertrophy and Right Ventricular dysfunction
↓ Vascular integrity with poor peripheral blood flow and hypertension
↑ Local and systemic inflammatory mediators
↑ Cellular injury in many, maybe all cells, including neurons

Maternal hyperglycemia produced dramatic adverse effects on fetal neural development.

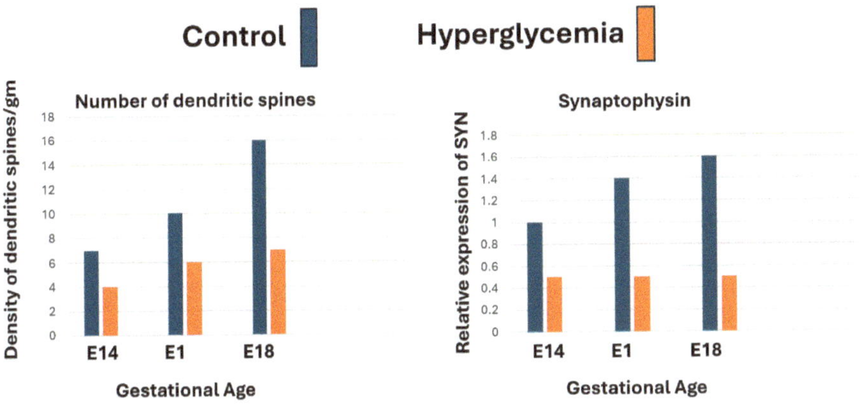

Maternal hyperglycemia restricted dendritic development in the fetal subplate cortex.

And reduced the expression of synaptophysin (SYN), a measure of synapse formation.

Fig. 8.8 Fetal hyperglycemia in hyperglycemic pregnant rats inhibits dendritic and synaptic development. (Adapted from: Jing et al. [41])

Adverse Fetal Neurodevelopmental Effects of Gestational Hyperglycemia

Chronic maternal and fetal hyperglycemia also produces dramatic adverse effects on fetal neural development. Animal models are notably convincing of such adverse effects. In a rat model of chronic gestational hyperglycemia, for example, maternal and thus fetal hyperglycemia restricts dendritic development in the fetal subplate cortex and reduces synaptophysin expression, a measure of synapse formation (Fig. 8.8) [41].

Mechanistically, chronic maternal hyperglycemia induced in mid-pregnancy in rats increases RAGE (Receptor for Advanced Glycation End-products), augments hippocampal excitability, and alters behavior of the offspring [42].

In humans, cognitive function is impaired in adolescent offspring of pregnant women with hyperglycemic type 1 diabetes vs. normoglycemic pregnant women. The impaired cognitive function is substantial, with highly significant lower intelligence indices including composite intelligence index, verbal intelligence index, nonverbal intelligence index, and composite memory index. Such individuals also display more learning difficulties, particularly with language and mathematics, but including reading and writing problems as well (Fig. 8.9) [43].

Adverse neurobehavioral and metabolic outcomes also were documented in a large, population-based cohort study in Ontario, Canada [44]. In this study, in utero exposure to maternal diabetes was associated with an increase in attention deficit hyperactivity disorder (ADHD), autism spectrum disorder, diabetes, and

Cognitive function is impaired in adolescent offspring of pregnant women with hyperglycemic type 1 diabetes (*n* = *277*) vs. normoglycemic pregnant women (*n* = *301*)

	Hyperglycemic	Normoglycemic	P value
Lower Intelligence Indices			
Composite Intelligence Index	95.7 (17.3)	100 (15)	0.001
Verbal Intelligence Index	96.2 (16.8)	100 (15)	0.004
Nonverbal Intelligence Index	96.4 (17)	100 (15	0.008
Composite Memory Index	95.7 (15.3)	100 (15)	0.001
More Learning Difficulties			
Reading Difficulties	22.4% (62)	18.7% (56)	0.269
Writing Difficulties	19.3% (52)	16.3% (48)	0.353
Learning Difficulties, Language	23.3% (64)	13.3% (41)	0.003
Learning Difficulties, Mathematics	16.4% (45)	7.7% (23)	0.001

Fig. 8.9 Prolonged fetal hyperglycemia in Type 1 diabetic pregnancies impairs cognitive function into adolescence. (Adapted from: Bytoft et al. [43])

cardiometabolic outcomes (hypertension, CVD) in the offspring. While clearly showing adverse effects of fetal hyperglycemia, this study also provides a potentially modifiable risk factor in pregnant women to decrease adverse neurological and cardiometabolic outcomes in offspring. A large meta-analysis also showed that maternal diabetes is associated with increased risks of all types of neurodevelopmental disorders as well as lower intelligence and psychomotor scores. In studies adjusting for multiple confounders (n = 98, 49%), children exposed to maternal diabetes had an increased risk of any neurodevelopmental disorder (risk ratio 1.28; 95% CI 1.24–1.31), autism spectrum disorder (1.25; 1.20–1.31), attention-deficit hyperactivity disorder (1.30; 1.24–1.37), intellectual disability (1.32; 1.18–1.47), specific developmental disorders (1.27; 1.17–1.37), communication disorder (1.20; 1.11–1.28), motor disorder (1.17; 1.10–1.26), and learning disorder (1.16; 1.06–1.26), compared with unexposed children. Maternal pre-gestational diabetes was more strongly associated with the risk of most neurodevelopmental disorders in children than gestational diabetes (risk ratio 1.39; [95% CI 1.34–1.44] *vs* 1.18 [1.14–1.23]; subgroup difference p < 0·0001), indicating that adverse effects of maternal diabetes with early gestational hyperglycemia during the early embryonic period could be particularly detrimental [45].

It remains unclear when during gestation hyperglycemia most affects cognitive development in the offspring and whether potentially adverse effects persist in adulthood. This problem was studied at the University of Cincinnati to determine the association between trimester-specific hyperglycemia exposure and adult cognition in the offspring of women with pregestational diabetes. The study included a comprehensive clinical examination and cognitive assessment (Wechsler Abbreviated Scale of Intelligence—II) to estimate the association between prenatal hyperglycemia and offspring's perceptual reasoning and verbal comprehension. The mean age at follow-up was 32.1 years. Hyperglycemia during pregnancy was inversely associated with cognitive measures, controlling for confounders including maternal education and pre-pregnancy obesity. Higher glycohemoglobin in the second and third trimesters was significantly linked to lower IQ scores, matrix reasoning, and vocabulary subtest scores in the adult offspring. Third-trimester hyperglycemia also was associated with lower "block design" subtest scores. These results emphasize that gestational hyperglycemia, particularly in the second half of pregnancy, may be associated with lower cognitive ability in adult offspring of women with pre-pregnancy pregestational diabetes [46].

Mechanisms for neuronal damage from hyperglycemia are not entirely clear, but in adults, astrocyte-endothelial signal transduction exposure to high glucose in diabetic conditions causes overproduction of vascular endothelial growth factor (VEGF) and abnormal proliferation of endothelial cells, loss of connexin 43 (Cx43) expression, cell membrane gap junctions, and astrocyte function, which correlate with the impairment in the blood-brain barrier [47]. Similar observations have been made in early developing astrocytes studied in culture [48].

Timing of Gestational Hyperglycemia and Effects on Offspring Metabolic and Body Fat Mass

Clearly, fetal hyperglycemia is common, largely due to maternal hyperglycemia (diabetes, obesity), and when chronic, makes the fetus fat, diminishes fetal insulin secretion, insulin action, and glucose uptake and utilization, especially in the IUGR fetus, as well as producing vascular, cardiac, and inflammatory cellular injuries, setting the stage for hyperglycemia and its complications in the neonate, infant, child, adolescent, and even the adult. In the case of later impacts on adult health, data are limited to convincingly demonstrate the long-term impact of pre-pregnancy diabetes on offspring body composition in adulthood. A recent study did, however, examine the association between maternal glucose control and variation throughout pregnancy and long-term risk of obesity in the offspring. This study also identified the critical windows of gestational exposure most related to the development of long-term obesity. Study participants included 32 year old adult offspring of women with insulin-dependent diabetes (IDDM). After adjustment for covariates (maternal age, education, family history of diabetes, diabetes severity, and BMI at last menstrual period), third-trimester maternal HbA1SD was significantly associated with offspring adiposity measures including BMI, BMI $\geq$30 kg/m^2, and visceral and whole-body fat mass and percentage. The third trimester demonstrated a consistent positive but borderline significant association between maternal HbA1SD with later obesity outcomes but did not reach statistical significance in adjusted models. The study overall, however, corroborated that the third trimester is a critical gestational period of excess fetal glucose exposure that is associated with offspring adiposity and that higher levels of third-trimester maternal glycohemoglobin A1 is a risk factor for obesity in the adult offspring of IDDM mothers. Additionally, results indicated that glucose variability may increase the risk for obesity in the adult offspring, consistent with the ovine fetal studies that showed increased fetal insulin secretion with variable, pulsatile, plasma glucose concentration excursions [49].

In contrast to these adverse offspring outcomes from late gestation maternal hyperglycemia, a recent study of relatively large magnitude (total of 4546 mother-child pairs) documented that GDM and impaired glucose tolerance, both with hyperglycemia, that were manifest in early pregnancy were associated with offspring neurodevelopmental delays (NDD) and autism spectrum disorder (ASD). These adverse outcomes were sex specific, documented significantly only in females. GDM overall and late gestation GDM with impaired glucose tolerance and hyperglycemia were not associated with increased odds of ASD (aOR, 1.15 [95% CI, 0.83–1.60]) or NDD (aOR, 1.24 [95% CI, 0.98–1.57]) [50].

Conclusions

Hyperglycemia in the fetus is directly related to maternal hyperglycemia, and when marked and sustained, produces many adverse outcomes. These can manifest in the fetus, persist in neonatal life, and contribute to risk for later life adverse outcomes in the offspring. Timing, however, is critical for some adverse outcomes of maternal hyperglycemic disorders, with early gestational hyperglycemia perhaps adversely producing neurological disorders in the offspring while cardiometabolic outcomes are associated more with later gestational hyperglycemia.

References

1. Marconi AM, Paolini C, Buscaglia M, Zerbe G, Battaglia FC, Pardi G. The impact of gestational age and fetal growth on the maternal-fetal glucose concentration difference. Obstet Gynecol. 1996;87:937–42.
2. Catalano PM. Carbohydrate metabolism and gestational diabetes. Clin Obstet Gynecol. 1994;37:25–38.
3. Shah NS, Wang MC, Freaney PM, Perak AM, Carnethon MR, Kandula NR, Gunderson EP, Bullard KM, Grobman WA, O'Brien MJ, Khan SS. Trends in gestational diabetes at first live birth by race and ethnicity in the US, 2011–2019. JAMA. 2021;326:660–9.
4. Lam EL, Walker JM, Wang MC, Venkatesh KK, Khan SS, Shah NS. Gestational diabetes in the US from 2016 to 2024. JAMA Intern Med 2026;186:269-271.
5. Kim SY, England L, Sappenfield W, Wilson HG, Bish CL, Salihu HM, Sharma AJ. Racial/ethnic differences in the percentage of gestational diabetes mellitus cases attributable to overweight and obesity, Florida, 2004–2007. Prev Chronic Dis. 2012;9:E88.
6. HAPO Study Cooperative Research Group, Metzger BE, Lowe LP, Dyer AR, Trimble ER, Chaovarindr U, Coustan DR, Hadden DR, McCance DR, Hod M, McIntyre HD, Oats JJ, Persson B, Rogers MS, Sacks DA. Hyperglycemia and adverse pregnancy outcomes. N Engl J Med. 2008;358:1991–2002.

7. Al Bekai E, Beaini CE, Kalout K, Safieddine O, Semaan S, Sahyoun F, Ghadieh HE, Azar S, Kanaan A, Harb F. The hidden impact of gestational diabetes: unveiling offspring complications and long-term effects. Life (Basel). 2025;15:440.
8. Shamsad A, Gautam T, Singh R, Banerjee M. Genetic and epigenetic alterations associated with gestational diabetes mellitus and adverse neonatal outcomes. World J Clin Pediatr. 2025;14:99231.
9. Das UG, Schroeder RE, Hay WW Jr, Devaskar SU. Time-dependent and tissue-specific effects of circulating glucose on fetal ovine glucose transporters. Am J Phys. 1999;276:R809–17.
10. Hay WW Jr, Meznarich HK. Use of fetal streptozotocin injection to determine the role of normal levels of fetal insulin in regulating uteroplacental and umbilical glucose exchange. Pediatr Res. 1988;24:312–27.
11. Hay WW Jr, Meznarich HK, Fowden A. The effects of streptozotocin on rates of glucose utilization, oxidation and production in the sheep fetus. Metabolism. 1988;38:30–7.
12. Carver TD, Anderson SM, Aldoretta PA, Esler AL, Hay WW Jr. Glucose suppression of insulin secretion in chronically hyperglycemic fetal sheep. Pediatr Res. 1995;38:754–62.
13. Hernandez TL, VanPelt RE, Anderson MA, Daniels LJ, West JA, Donahoo WT, Friedman JE, Barbour LA. A higher complex carbohydrate diet in gestational diabetes achieves glucose targets and lowers postprandial lipids: a randomized crossover study. Diabetes Care. 2014;37:1254–62.
14. Hernandez TL, Farab SS, Van Pelt RE, Hirsch N, Dunn EZ, Haugen EA, Reece MS, Friedman JE, Barbour LA. Continuous glucose monitor metrics that predict neonatal adiposity early and later pregnancy are higher in obesity despite macronutrient controlled, eucaloric diets. Nutrients. 2024;16:3489.
15. Hay WW Jr. Recent observations on the regulation of fetal metabolism by glucose. J Physiol. 2006;572:17–24.
16. Carver TD, Anderson SM, Aldoretta PW, Hay WW Jr. Effect of low-level basal plus marked "pulsatile" hyperglycemia on insulin secretion in fetal sheep. Am J Phys. 1996;271:E865–71.
17. Nicolini U, Hubinont C, Santolaya J, Fisk NM, Rodeck CH. Effects of fetal intravenous glucose challenge in normal and growth retarded fetuses. Horm Metab Res. 1990;22:426–30.
18. Brereton MF, Rohm M, Shimomura K, Holland C, Tornovsky-Babeay S, Dadon D, Iberl M, Chibalina MV, Lee S, Glaser B, Dor Y, Rorsman P, Clark A, Ashcroft FM. Hyperglycaemia induces metabolic dysfunction and glycogen accumulation in pancreatic β-cells. Nat Commun. 2016;7:13496.
19. Limesand SW, Rozance PJ, Zerbe GO, Hutton JC, Hay WW Jr. Attenuated insulin release and storage in fetal sheep pancreatic islets with intrauterine growth restriction. Endocrinology. 2006;14:1488–97.
20. Andrews SE, Brown LD, Thorn SR, Limesand SW, Davis M, Hay WW Jr, Rozance PJ. Increased adrenergic signaling is responsible for decreased glucose-stimulated insulin secretion in the chronically hyperinsulinemic ovine fetus. Endocrinology. 2015;156:367–76.
21. Leos RA, Anderson MJ, Chen X, Pugmire J, Anderson KA, Limesand SW. Chronic exposure to elevated norepinephrine suppresses insulin secretion in fetal sheep with placental insufficiency and intrauterine growth restriction. Am J Physiol Endocrinol Metab. 2010;298:E770–8.
22. Cilvik SN, Boehmer B, Wesolowski SR, Brown LD, Rozance PJ. Chronic late gestation fetal hyperglucagonaemia results in lower insulin secretion, pancreatic mass, islet area, and beta- and α-cell proliferation. J Physiol. 2024;602:6329–45.
23. Lewandowski SL, El K, Campbell JE. Evaluating glucose-dependent insulinotropic polypeptide and glucagon as key regulators of insulin secretion in the pancreatic islet. Am J Physiol Endocrinol Metab. 2024;327:E103–10.
24. Eisenstein AB, Strack I. Amino acid stimulation of glucagon secretion by perifused islets of high-protein-fed rats. Diabetes. 1978;27:370–6.
25. Kuhara T, Ikeda S, Ohneda A, Sasaki Y. Effects of intravenous infusion of 17 amino acids on the secretion of Gh, glucagon, and insulin in sheep. Am J Phys. 1991;260:E21–6.

26. Galsgaard KD, Jepsen SL, Kjeldsen SAS, Pedersen J, Wewer Albrechtsen NJ, Holst JJ. Alanine, arginine, cysteine, and proline, but not glutamine, are substrates for, and acute mediators of, the liver-α-cell axis in female mice. Am J Physiol Endocrinol Metab. 2020;318:E920–9.
27. Guiducci S, Res G, Bonadies L, Savio F, Brigadoi S, Priante E, Trevisanuto D, Baraldi E, Galderisi A. Impact of macronutrients intake on glycemic homeostasis of preterm infants: evidence from continuous glucose monitoring. Eur J Pediatr. 2024;183:3013–8.
28. Larsson H, Ahren B. Glucose-dependent arginine stimulation test for characterization of islet function: studies on reproducibility and priming effect of arginine. Diabetologia. 1998;41:772–7.
29. Sunehag A, Ewald U, Gustafsson J. Extremely preterm infants (< 28 weeks) are capable of gluconeogenesis from glycerol on their first day of life. Pediatr Res. 1996;40:553–7.
30. Sunehag AL. The role of parenteral lipids in supporting gluconeogenesis in very premature infants. Pediatr Res. 2003;54:480–6.
31. Sunehag AL. Parenteral glycerol enhances gluconeogenesis in very premature infants. Pediatr Res. 2003;53:635–41.
32. Chacko SK, Sunehag AL. Gluconeogenesis continues in premature infants receiving total parenteral nutrition. Arch Dis Child Fetal Neonatal Ed. 2010;95:F413–8.
33. Salle BL, Ruiton-Ugliengo A. Effects of oral glucose and protein load on plasma glucagon and insulin concentrations in small for gestational age infants. Pediatr Res. 1977;11:108–12.
34. Limesand SW, Rozance PJ. Fetal adaptations in insulin secretion result from high catecholamines during placental insufficiency. J Physiol. 2017;595:5103–13.
35. Wesolowski SR, Hay WW Jr. Role of placental insufficiency and intrauterine growth restriction on the activation of fetal hepatic glucose production. Mol Cell Endocrinol. 2016;435:61–8.
36. Thorn SR, Brown LD, Rozance PJ, Hay WW Jr, Friedman JE. Increased hepatic glucose production in fetal sheep with intrauterine growth restriction is not suppressed by insulin. Diabetes. 2013;62:65–73.
37. Thorn SR, Regnault TR, Brown LD, Rozance PJ, Keng J, Roper M, Wilkening RB, Hay WW Jr, Friedman JE. Intrauterine growth restriction increases fetal hepatic gluconeogenic capacity and reduces messenger ribonucleic acid translation initiation and nutrient sensing in fetal liver and skeletal muscle. Endocrinology. 2009;150:3021–30.
38. Durga KD, Adhisivam B, Vidya G, Vishnu Bhat B, Bobby Z, Chand P. Oxidative stress and DNA damage in newborns born to mothers with hyperglycemia – a prospective cohort study. J Matern Fetal Neonatal Med. 2018;31:2396–401.
39. Guleria RS, Pan J, Dipette D, Singh US. Hyperglycemia inhibits retinoic acid-induced activation of Rac1, prevents differentiation of cortical neurons, and causes oxidative stress in a rat model of diabetic pregnancy. Diabetes. 2006;55:3326–33.
40. Michelsen TM, Sajjad MU, Haugen G, Moore L, Julian CG, Sørbye IK, Henriksen T. Maternal body mass index is related to fetal uptake of glucose and oxygen via fetal insulin resistance rather than fetal glucose levels. Philos Trans R Soc Lond Ser B Biol Sci. 2025;380(1933):20240178.
41. Jing YH, Song YF, Yao YM, Yin J, Wang DG, Gao LP. Retardation of fetal dendritic development induced by gestational hyperglycemia is associated with brain insulin/IGF-I signals. Int J Dev Neurosci. 2014;37:15–20.
42. Campanucci VA, Howland JG. Chronic maternal hyperglycemia induced during mid-pregnancy in rats increases RAGE expression, augments hippocampal excitability, and alters behavior of the offspring. Neuroscience. 2015;303:241–60.
43. Bytoft B, Knorr S, Vlachova Z, Jensen RB, Mathiesen ER, Beck-Nielsen H, Gravholt CH, Jensen DM, Clausen TD, Mortensen EL, Damm P. Long-term cognitive implications of intrauterine hyperglycemia in adolescent offspring of women with type 1 diabetes (the EPICOM study). Diabetes Care. 2016;39:1356–63.
44. Feig DS, Artani A, Asaf A, Li P, Booth GL, Shah BR. Long-term neurobehavioral and metabolic outcomes in offspring of mothers with diabetes during pregnancy: a large, population-based cohort study in Ontario, Canada. Diabetes Care. 2024;47:1568–75.

45. Ye W, Luo C, Zhou J, Liang X, Wen J, Huang J, Zeng Y, Wu Y, Gao Y, Liu Z, Liu F. Association between maternal diabetes and neurodevelopmental outcomes in children: a systematic review and meta-analysis of 202 observational studies comprising 56·1 million pregnancies. Lancet Diabetes Endocrinol. 2025;13:494–504.
46. Bowers K, Yolton K, Catalano P, Khoury JC. Association between maternal glycohemoglobin in pregnancy and adult offspring cognition: results from the Transgenerational Effects of Adult Morbidity (TEAM) Study. J Dev Orig Health Dis. 2025;16:e26.
47. Garvin J, Semenikhina M, Liu Q, Rarick K, Isaeva E, Levchenko V, Staruschenko A, Palygin O, Harder D, Cohen S. Astrocytic responses to high glucose impair barrier formation in cerebral microvessel endothelial cells. Am J Physiol Regul Integr Comp Physiol. 2022;322:R571–80.
48. Cohen S, Liu Q, Wright M, Garvin J, Rarick K, Harder D. High glucose conditioned neonatal astrocytes results in impaired mitogenic activity in cerebral microvessel endothelial cells in co-culture. Heliyon. 2019;5:e01795.
49. Bowers K, Bhoopathy KK, Szczesniak R, Ehrlich S, Dolan LM, Kalkwarf H, Summer S, Smith E, Altaye M, Ollberding NJ, Catalano P, Miodovnik M, Khoury JC. Timing and variability of maternal hyperglycemia in insulin-dependent diabetes, long-term effects on offspring obesity—the TEAM study. Pregnancy. 2025;1:e70048.
50. Grosvenor LP, Gunderson EP, Qian Y, Alexeeff S, Ames JL, Weiss LA, Sahagun E, Ashwood P, Yolken R, Zhu Y, Van de Water J, Croen LA. Prenatal glucose intolerance and child neurodevelopmental disorders. JAMA Netw Open. 2025;8:e2541657.

Chapter 9
Evidence for and Definitions of Normal and Abnormal High Glucose Concentrations

William W. Hay, Jr.

Risk Factors for Neonatal Hyperglycemia

First, what is "Neonatal Hyperglycemia"? Unfortunately, there are no reported clinical definitions or clinical signs specific to hyperglycemia (i.e., the appearance of physiological disturbances associated with a specific high blood or plasma glucose concentration). Some reviews, however, refer to older and non-specific clinical signs such as polyuria, dehydration, acidosis, failure to thrive, and poor weight gain, tachypnea, blood oxygen desaturations, altered sensorium, or stroke with progression to diabetic ketoacidosis [1, 2]. Most of these are signs of conditions that simply are associated with hyperglycemia [3].

Frequent and prolonged hyperglycemic events are, however, associated with significant sequelae, even if evidence for causality is lacking. In addition, the lack of standardization in the definition criteria and the wide variations in the management of hyperglycemia have caused further confusion about the actual role of hyperglycemic events in the development of neonatal mortality and morbidity [4]. One must, therefore, measure plasma glucose concentrations to see if hyperglycemia is present. Definition thresholds for hyperglycemia vary significantly in the literature and range from 125 to more than 180 mg/dL (>7 to >10 mmol/L). The duration of hyperglycemia and the association with glycosuria have also been assessed. Plasma glucose concentration >150 mg/dL (>8.3 mmol/L), appears to be the starting threshold for developing glycosuria in VLBW infants [5]. In addition, outcomes associated with hyperglycemia are reported by differences in severity or number of episodes of hyperglycemia.

W. W. Hay, Jr. (✉)
University of Colorado, Denver, CO, USA
e-mail: bill.hay@ucdenver.edu

D. H. Adamkin, W. W. Hay, Jr. (eds.), *Disorders of Neonatal Glycemia*,
https://doi.org/10.1007/978-3-032-29094-6_9

Definition of Neonatal Hyperglycemia

In textbooks: many authors arbitrarily define neonatal hyperglycemia as >125 mg/dL blood (>150 mg/dL plasma (>7 mmol/L blood, >8.4 mmol/L plasma) in a term infant, but slightly higher at about 150 mg/dL blood (175 mg/dL plasma) in preterm infants [6]. Most neonatologists polled, however, have defined hyperglycemia threshold blood concentration as not clinically significant until >180 mg/dL (>10 mmol/L) [7]. Definition thresholds differ from intervention thresholds, and a glucose cutoff of 180 mg/dL (10.0 mmol/L) has been suggested as a starting point for treatment consideration [8]. In truth, there is no clinically relevant data to support any one of these definitions. There is no justification not to accept a value of 108 mg/dL (6 mmol/L) as the upper limit of normal glucose concentrations as occur in the normal healthy fetus in later gestation and similar values in normal term infants and children.

Neonatal hyperglycemia is rare in term infants unless they are receiving high rate IV dextrose infusions. It most commonly occurs in preterm infants and is inversely related to gestational age at birth, and particularly those with low birth weight and IUGR [9–11], and during the first week or so of postnatal life, although it can persist for many days, especially in infants who had IUGR [4, 12, 13]. Such infants almost always receive IV dextrose infusions aimed at preventing hypoglycemia and as part of parenteral nutrition. Hyperglycemia also can persist over the first month of life, potentially leading to underestimation of its incidence, duration, and relationship to pathological conditions in studies that have focused on early monitoring. Clinically stable VLBW infants on full enteral bolus feeds can be at risk for hyperglycemia for up to 8 weeks of life [14–17] Given the lack of data over longer periods and the multitude of associated disorders that preterm infants experience, the significance of such events remains unknown. Variations in glucose levels, rather than actual hyperglycemia, might be more important in the immediate mortality and morbidity in VLBW preterm infants; Hyperglycemia in VLBW infants in the first week was also found to be associated with increased mortality [18].

What Causes Neonatal Hyperglycemia?

Table 9.1 identifies the most common causes of neonatal hyperglycemia. In one large study, 66/859 (8%) infants ≤32 weeks of gestation developed hyperglycemia. Mortality during admission was 27/66 (41%) in the hyperglycemia group versus 62/793 (8%) in those without hyperglycemia ($p < 0.001$). Mortality was higher in infants with hyperglycemia with a birth weight ≤1000 g ($p = 0.005$) and/or gestational age of 24–28 weeks ($p = 0.009$) than in control infants without hyperglycemia. Sepsis was more prominent in infants with hyperglycemia and a birth weight of >1000 g ($p = 0.002$) and/or gestational age of 29–32 weeks ($p = 0.009$) than in control infants without hyperglycemia. Growth at 2 years of age was similar, but

Table 9.1 Etiology of neonatal hyperglycemia

1. **Preterm birth and Intrauterine growth restriction**
Inadequate insulin secretion and inability to suppress glucose production in the liver
Increased insulin resistance
2. **Increased stress hormones** like epinephrine and norepinephrine inhibit both insulin secretion and action. They also increase glucagon, which promotes glycogenolysis. The following conditions are associated with increased stress hormones
Catecholamine infusions
Seizures
Physiological stress caused by surgery, pain, hypoxia, respiratory distress, or sepsis
3. **Causes related to enteral feeding**
A delay in the initiation of enteral feeding causes decreased incretin secretion, which in turn causes hyperglycemia [19].
The hyperosmolar formula may lead to transient glucose intolerance in the infant.
4. **Causes related to total parenteral nutrition (TPN)**
A delay in supplementing parenteral amino acids in TPN delays the release of insulin-like growth factor-1, which delays the development of beta cells in the pancreas and develops hyperglycemia.
A high intravenous lipid infusion rate causes an increase in free fatty acids, which decrease glucose oxidation competitively by providing additional carbon substrates for oxidative metabolism. Free fatty acids and glycerol promote gluconeogenesis [20].
5. **Sepsis**: Consider sepsis and necrotizing enterocolitis if hyperglycemia develops without a change in glucose infusion rate.
6. **Iatrogenic**: An all too common causes of hyperglycemia in the neonate is an error in the glucose infusion rate (GIR) calculation in the intravenous (IV) fluids, or a pharmacy error in accidentally using D75 for infusion when it usually is used as an additive to D5 to produce, for example, D7.5, or to D10 to produce D12.5. The highest infusate dextrose concentration in the author's personal experience was 2950 mg/dL (164 mmol/L) that caused severe osmotic intracranial hemorrhage [21].
7. **Transient neonatal diabetes mellitus** usually occurs in small for gestational age infants. This condition is self-limited.
8. **Drugs**
Maternal medications
Maternal diazoxide may cause hyperglycemia, hypotension, and tachycardia in neonates.
Antenatal steroids
Neonatal medications
Dopamine, dobutamine, epinephrine infusions
Caffeine, theophylline
Phenytoin
Corticosteroids

Adapted from: Balasundaram and Dumpa [22], Hay Jr. and Rozance [19], and Rozance and Hay Jr. [21]

neurological and behavioral development was more frequently abnormal among those with neonatal hyperglycemia ($p = 0.036$ and 0.021 respectively) [23]. Hyperglycemia was most common among preterm infants <28 weeks (50%). Female gender increased the chances of developing hypoglycemia by three times.

The decrease in gestational age by 1 week increased the chance of developing hyperglycemia by 1.9 times. Sepsis increased the chance of developing hyperglycemia seven times, respiratory distress syndrome five times, and mechanical ventilation three times, respectively [24].

Hyperglycemia and Metabolic Immaturity

Hyperglycemia often has been attributed to immaturity in several cellular pathways involved in glucose metabolism in preterm infants, especially those born very early and frequently with IUGR. Certain nutritional deficiencies also can lead to hyperglycemia. For example, preterm infants have low zinc concentrations, which have been associated with hyperglycemia. There is a strong physiological link between zinc and glycemic control, although this has been mainly observed in adults with diabetes. Zinc plays an important role in insulin secretion. Zinc can enhance the phosphorylation of insulin receptors and intracellular signaling, and the translocation of glucose transporter 4 (GLUT4) to the plasma membrane, which increases cellular uptake of glucose in response to insulin. Data that directly link serum zinc concentration to hyperglycemia are lacking in preterm newborns, although adding zinc, which has been used increasingly in recent years to promote growth, might counter the effect of zinc deficiency, as zinc increases glycogen synthesis and inhibits gluconeogenesis. In one study of appropriate for GA (AGA), 23–28-week GA infants, increasing the dose of zinc in parenteral fluid from 300 to 450 mcg/kg/day, without changing the average energy or protein intake, was followed by a decrease in the number of glucose POC values >150 mg/dL (8.33 mmol/L) from a median of 2 (interquartile range [IQR] 0.14) to 1 (IQR 0.6) ($P = 0.006$), while the number of hypoglycemic values did not change [4].

Similarly, there is good evidence that other factors contribute to glucose tolerance and risk of hyperglycemia. For example, adding chromium to parenteral nutrition therapy in preterm infants (0.2 μg/kg/day) can increase glucose tolerance and reduce glucose concentrations and the incidence and severity of hyperglycemia. Chromium potentiates insulin action [25]. Arginine also potentiates inulin action and its concentration in TPN solutions is low. Low plasma arginine concentrations (≤57 μmol/L) have been associated with increased insulin-treated hyperglycemia and higher mean daily blood glucose levels in very preterm infants [26].

Preterm infants have lower levels of insulin and demonstrate peripheral insulin resistance. They also have reduced muscle mass that limits glucose utilization—only about 10% of whole body glucose utilization is insulin dependent [27–30]. Rarely, neonatal hyperglycemia is related to congenital monogenic diabetes [31].

Primary Adverse Contributions to Hyperglycemia from High IV Dextrose Infusion Rates

A primary cause of hyperglycemia has been the fear of hypoglycemia that has led to the common approach of starting high to excessively high IV glucose (dextrose) infusion rates, often as high as 6–8 mg/min/kg, that are commonly started right after birth, increasing to 12–14 mg/min/kg for full intravenous nutrition (IVN). Intravenous nutrition in preterm infants has become universal, especially in the first few days after birth before full enteral nutrition is established [32]. Early, full IVN and high rates of IV dextrose infusions, however, have become common practice sort of reflexively, without considering that most of these infants are already at risk of hyperglycemia. Such risk is in part due to fetal conditions that promote glucose production and reduce glucose and insulin sensitivity. It also is the result of neonatal illnesses or other pathophysiology and treatments that promote glucose production, reduce insulin secretion and plasma concentrations, and raise glucose concentrations.

Excess IV dextrose infusion rates also ignore the fact that maximal glucose utilization rates (GUR) normally are lower than assumed. For preterm infants ~28 weeks gestation, for example, glucose utilization has been measured by stable isotope methodology at about 5–7 mg/min/kg GUR, largely for the brain but also the heart. By term gestation, glucose utilization rates have declined to about 3–5 mg/min/kg GUR, still largely brain and heart, but lower per kg body weight than earlier in gestation due to growth of fat, skeletal muscle, skin, bone, lung, and GI track tissues that have low GURs [33]. And with early and/or prolonged TPN, the actual intake of nutrients has been weighted to energy, carbohydrate (mostly glucose) and lipid (mostly fatty acids and glycerol), but less protein and its stimulation of insulin secretion, which together promote hyperglycemia (Fig. 9.1) [34].

Higher than needed rates of IV glucose infusion compound other risks for hyperglycemia in neonates. Preterm birth, low birthweight, and IUGR are associated with less insulin secretion, with fewer pancreatic islets and β-cells, and when persistent

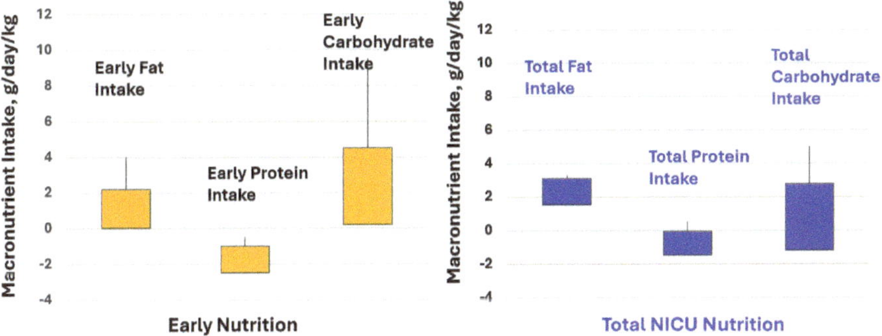

Fig. 9.1 Early and total NICU fat, protein, and carbohydrate intake in preterm infants receiving intravenous nutrition. (Adapted from: Vasu et al. [34])

due to stress after birth as studied in fetal and neonatal sheep, suppression of glucose stimulated insulin secretion by catecholamines [35, 36]. The absence of enteral feeding also prevents or limits secretion of GI tract incretins, proteins that already are low in preterm ELBW infants. Incretins are absorbed into the circulation from the GI tract and promote pancreatic insulin secretion.

Contributions of Persistent Glucose Production

Early and high rates of IV lipid infusion promote hepatic glucose production (GPR) and reduce glucose utilization. Intermittent hypoxia promotes production of catecholamines and cortisol that promote hepatic GPR and insulin resistance in peripheral tissues. The same actions occur with the infusion of catecholamines [37] and/or steroids such as hydrocortisone and Decadron [38, 39]. There also is postnatal persistence of increased endogenous hepatic glucose production rate (EhGPR) in preterm infants, especially those with IUGR, due to continued increased hepatic insulin resistance that promotes persistent EhGPR [40, 41]. It is likely that IUGR is central in this pathological condition, as not all studies have shown that preterm infants continue hepatic GPR at lower glucose concentrations [42].

Of particular note, however, EPT/ELBW hyperglycemic preterm neonates (particularly those with IUGR) can have unsuppressed EhGPR at a much higher blood glucose range than commonly documented in the literature (Fig. 9.2). Furthermore, EhGPR) in these infants is relatively independent of birth weight and gestational age [43].

As a direct result, neonatal plasma and blood glucose concentrations increase directly and linearly with any increase in IV glucose infusion rate, because glucose

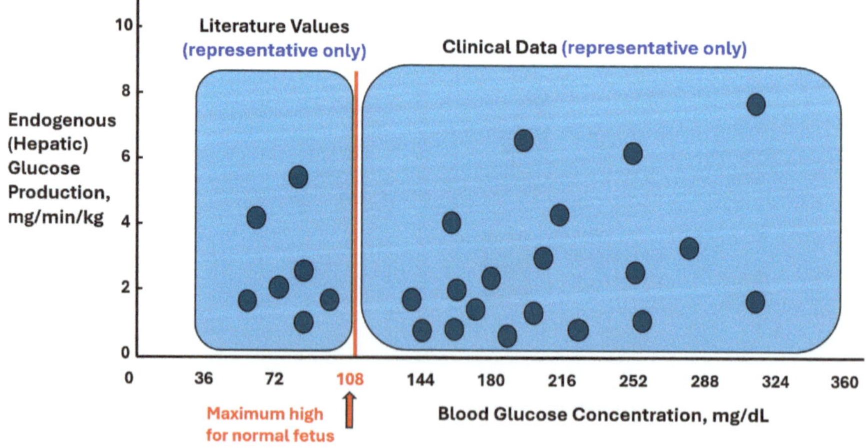

Fig. 9.2 Endogenous glucose production in neonates. (Adapted from: Dickson et al. [43])

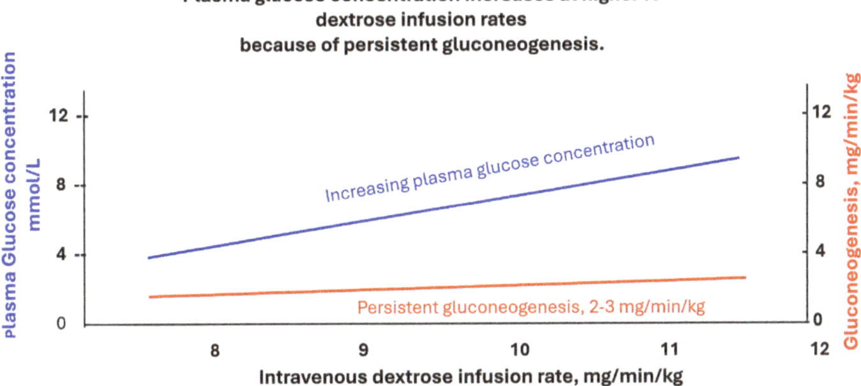

Fig. 9.3 Gluconeogenesis persists in preterm infants after birth, augmenting glucose excess from IV nutrition. (Adapted from: Chacko and Sunehag [44])

production persists in newborns (2–3 mg/kg/min), especially preterm and IUGR infants, despite high glucose and insulin concentrations (Fig. 9.3) [44].

Risk for hyperglycemia from glucose production is further compounded by glucagon secretion, normally produced at birth but increased from stress. Glucagon promotes glycogenolysis (activates glycogen phosphorylase) and gluconeogenesis (activates PEPCK, especially when insulin is low) [45–48]. FFAs also competitively limit glucose oxidation. This reduces the capacity for glucose and insulin to increase cellular glucose uptake and utilization, thus inhibiting their effects to decrease plasma glucose.

Intermittent hypoxic-ischemic conditions that are common after preterm birth lead to increased secretion of counter-regulatory hormones (catecholamines, cortisol) that produce hyperglycemia by increasing glycogenolysis, decreasing insulin secretion and insulin action, increasing protein breakdown that releases gluconeogenic amino acids, and increased gluconeogenesis [21, 49]. The effect of catecholamines on reducing insulin production is particularly profound. Experiments in fetal sheep have shown a >2-fold reduction in glucose stimulated insulin secretion at plasma adrenalin concentrations similar to those produced by acute hypoxia [50].

Preterm Birth and Metabolic Immaturity

Hyperglycemia is common in very low-birthweight infants, more so in the most preterm infants (Fig. 9.4) [51, 52].

In a careful prospective observational cohort study of repeated glucose concentration measurements in preterm infants in Umeå, Sweden, hyperglycemia >10 mmol/L was found in 63% of 49 VLBW infants. Hyperglycemia occurred most commonly in the first week after birth. While hyperglycemia followed 15% of

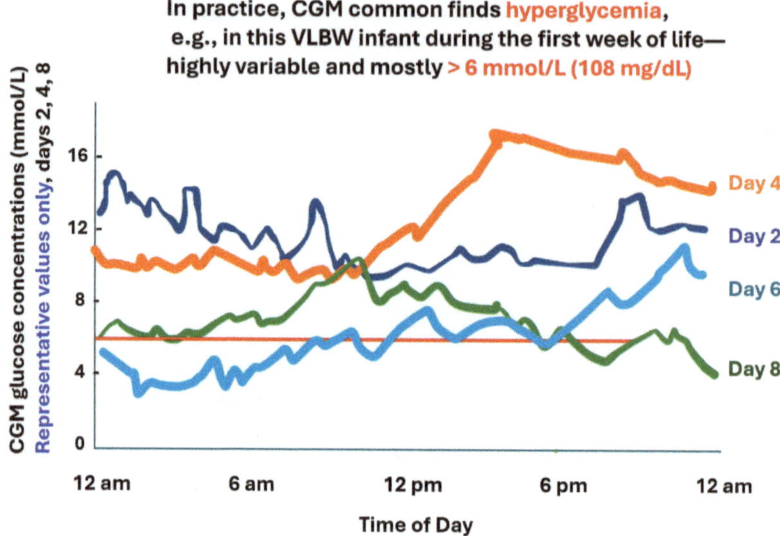

Fig. 9.4 Continuous glucose monitoring of plasma glucose concentrations in a VLBW preterm infant over 1 day. (Adapted from: Ogilvy-Stuart and Beardsall [51])

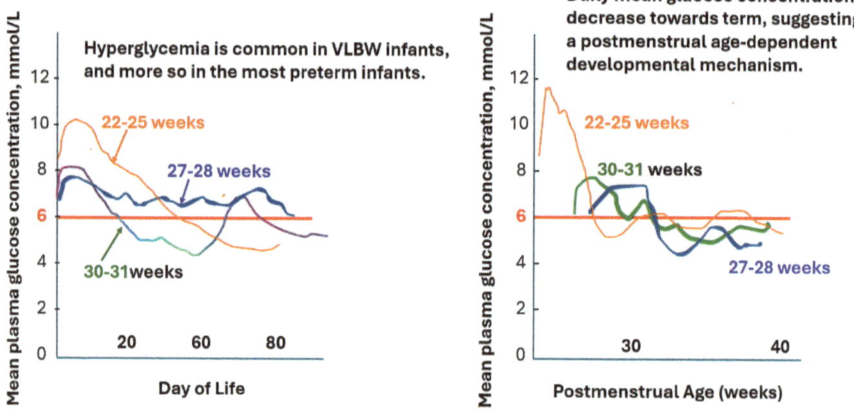

Fig. 9.5 Early postnatal hyperglycemia is common in preterm infants but declines with gestational age. (Adapted from: Zamir et al. [53])

corticosteroid doses and 67% of inotrope treatments, all had pre-existing hyperglycemia. At least in this study, initial hyperglycemia was independent of sepsis and corticosteroid and inotrope treatments, but these conditions and treatments were noted to prolong hyperglycemia. Furthermore, as shown in Fig. 9.5, daily mean glucose concentrations decrease towards term age indicating a postmenstrual age-dependent developmental mechanism [53].

Nevertheless, corticosteroid administration can have profound and dose dependent increases in glucose concentration by promoting glucose production and release from glycogen and hepatocytes and from inhibiting insulin secretion and action. Standard high doses of steroids have been shown to production glucose concentration as high as 1000–1800 mg/dL, which easily could be damaging to neurons, especially if prolonged or repeated [54].

While not generally measured (only by careful MRI research studies that still lack verification), preterm and especially IUGR infants have relatively lower amounts of insulin-sensitive tissues (e.g., skeletal muscle and heart) as a fraction of body weight, which will manifest as lower weight-specific glucose utilization rates. Interestingly, the reduced skeletal muscle mass in preterm and IUGR infants can persist throughout infancy and childhood and even into adulthood and has been associated with reduced body weight specific insulin action and glucose [55]. Preterm and IUGR infants also may have abnormal pancreatic β-cell insulin processing that produces relatively more immature forms of insulin (proinsulin and proinsulin split products). These immature forms of insulin are less effective in binding with the insulin receptors, thus contributing to relative insulin resistance [56]. Insulin resistance also is simply more common in preterm infants, even in the absence of hyperglycemia, and despite increased glucagon-like peptide-1 (GLP-1) enteral feedings that ordinarily would cause an increase in insulin secretion [57].

Contributions of IV Nutrition, Particularly Total Intravenous Nutrition (TPN)

There is increasing evidence that Intravenous feeding or total parenteral nutrition (TPN) in neonates leads to insulin resistance that initially increases insulin production, but also glucose Intolerance via down-regulation of glucose transporters. Prolonged TPN, still common in preterm infants, especially those born extremely preterm with extremely low birth weight, and as shown in neonatal piglets, can lead to reduced proliferating insulin-producing pancreatic β-cells, decreased insulin-positive cells as a fraction of total pancreatic cells, and decreased proliferating pancreatic β-cells as a fraction of total Insulin containing cells. These changes in response to hyperglycemia eventually will limit the initial increase in pancreatic insulin secretion in response to insulin resistance [58]. In the same piglet studies, there also is evidence that prolonged TPN reduces relative abundance and activation of proteins that regulate insulin action in liver and skeletal muscle (insulin receptor, insulin receptor substrate, and PI3-kinase). Together, while clearly shown in an animal model, prolonged TPN, perhaps due to maintained higher than normal glucose concentrations, can promote insulin resistance leading to persistent hyperglycemia, or at least higher than normal glucose concentrations.

High glucose concentrations also trigger a series of metabolic pathway mediators within vascular smooth muscle cells that increase arterial myogenic tone,

Increasing dextrose infusion rates over the first week of life in preterm infants has resulted in a marked increase in the incidence of severe hyperglycemic episodes.

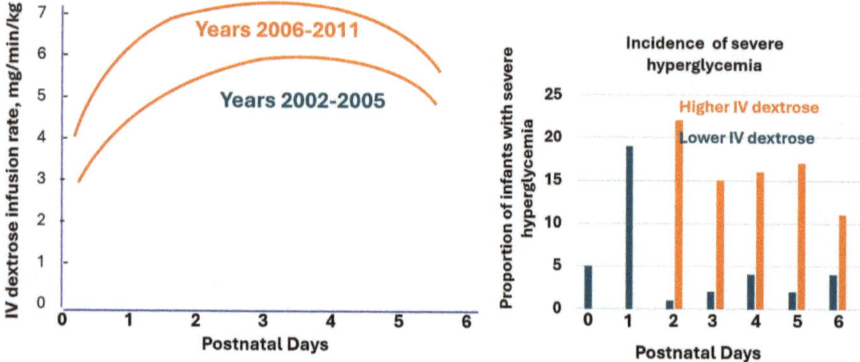

Fig. 9.6 Increased IV dextrose infusions and total carbohydrate and calorie intake have produced severe hyperglycemia. (Adapted from: Stensvold et al. [12])

reduce tissue blood flow, and promote hypertension [59]. This may be due to glucose or to secondary increases in insulin secretion and insulin concentrations in the circulation. The latter has been proposed as an underlying mechanism for neonatal cardiac hypertrophy that is commonly seen in infants of diabetic mothers [60].

As a result of these many conditions that predispose preterm infants to higher-than-normal glucose concentrations, decreased glucose stimulated insulin secretion, and insulin resistance, neonatal hyperglycemia in preterm and especially IUGR infants have become increasingly common, perhaps universal (Fig. 9.6) [12].

Conclusions

Overall, neonatal hyperglycemia is common, particularly in EPT to VPT, ELBW to VLBW and commonly IUGR infants, largely due to excess dextrose infusion, compounded by many conditions starting in the fetus and developing after birth that increase risks of hyperglycemia, and it gets worse the longer it persists.

References

1. Hemachandra AH, Cowett RM. Neonatal hyperglycemia. Pediatr Rev. 1999;20:e16–24.
2. Hey E. Hyperglycaemia and the very preterm baby. Semin Fetal Neonatal Med. 2005;10:377–87.
3. Lagacé M, Tam EWY. Neonatal dysglycemia: a review of dysglycemia in relation to brain health and neurodevelopmental outcomes. Pediatr Res. 2024;96:1429–37.
4. Angelis D, Jaleel MA, Brion LP. Hyperglycemia and prematurity: a narrative review. Pediatr Res. 2023;94:892–903.

5. Jagla M, Szymonska I, Starzec K, Kwinta P. Preterm glycosuria-new data from a continuous glucose monitoring system. Neonatology. 2018;114:87–92.
6. Rozance PJ, McGowan JE, Price-Douglas W, Hay WW Jr. Chapter 15, Glucose homeostasis. In: Gardner SL, Carter BS, Enzman-Hines M, Niermeyer S, editors. Neonatal intensive care. 9th ed. St. Louis: Elsevier; 2020. p. 431–58.
7. Alsweiler JM, Kuschel CA, Bloomfield FH. Survey of the management of neonatal hyperglycaemia in Australasia. J Paediatr Child Health. 2007;43:632–5.
8. Mesotten D, Joosten K, van Kempen A, Verbruggen S. ESPGHAN/ESPEN/ESPR/CSPEN working group on pediatric parenteral nutrition ESPGHAN/ESPEN/ESPR/CSPEN guidelines on pediatric parenteral nutrition: carbohydrates. Clin Nutr. 2018;37:2337–43.
9. Ramel S, Rao R. Hyperglycemia in extremely preterm infants. NeoReviews. 2020;21(2):e89–97.
10. Blanco CL, Baillargeon JG, Morrison RL, Gong AK. Hyperglycemia in extremely low birth weight infants in a predominantly hispanic population and related morbidities. J Perinatol. 2006;26:737–41.
11. Beardsall K, Vanhaesebrouck S, Ogilvy-Stuart AL, Vanhole C, Palmer CR, Ong K, vanWeissenbruch M, Midgley P, Thompson M, Thio M, Cornette L, Ossuetta I, Iglesias I, Theyskens C, de Jong M, Gill B, Ahluwalia JS, de Zegher F, Dunger DB. Prevalence and determinants of hyperglycemia in very low birth weight infants: cohort analyses of the NIRTURE study. J Pediatr. 2010;157:715–7.
12. Stensvold HJ, Strommen K, Lang AM, Abrahamsen TG, Steen EK, Pripp AH, Ronnestad AE. Early enhanced parenteral nutrition, hyperglycemia, and death among extremely low-birth-weight infants. JAMA Pediatr. 2015;169:1003–10.
13. Szymońska I, Jagła M, Starzec K, Hrnciar K, Kwinta P. The incidence of hyperglycaemia in very low birth weight preterm newborns. Results of a continuous glucose monitoring study—preliminary report. Dev Period Med. 2015;19:305–12.
14. Pertierra-Cortada A, Ramon-Krauel M, Iriondo-Sanz M, Iglesias-Platas I. Instability of glucose values in very preterm babies at term postmenstrual age. J Pediatr. 2014;165:1146–1153.e1142.
15. Mola-Schenzle E, Staffler A, Klemme M, Pellegrini F, Molinaro G, Parhofer KG, Messner H, Schulze A, Flemmer AW. Clinically stable very low birthweight infants are at risk for recurrent tissue glucose fluctuations even after fully established enteral nutrition. Arch Dis Child Fetal Neonatal Ed. 2015;100:F126–31.
16. Dina Mohammed Akmal DM, Abdel Rahman Ahmed Abdel Razek ARAA, Noha Musa N, El-Aziz AGA. Incidence, risk factors and complications of hyperglycemia in very low birth weight infants. Egypt Pediatr Assoc Gaz. 2017;65:72–9.
17. Saputri S, Alodia B, Habiburrahman M. Neonatal hyperglycaemia in extremely preterm and extremely low birth weight infants: a report of a rare case and a review of the literature. World Acad Sci J. 2024;6:37.
18. Mizumoto H, Kawai M, Yamashita S, Hata D. Intraday glucose fluctuation is common in preterm infants receiving intermittent tube feeding. Pediatr Int. 2016;58:359–62.
19. Hay WW Jr, Rozance PJ. Neonatal hyperglycemia-causes, treatments, and cautions. J Pediatr. 2018;200:6–8.
20. Vileisis RA, Cowett RM, Oh W. Glycemic response to lipid infusion in the premature neonate. J Pediatr. 1982;100:108–12.
21. Rozance PJ, Hay WW Jr. Neonatal hyperglycemia. NeoReviews. 2010;11:e632.
22. Balasundaram P, Dumpa V. Neonatal hyperglycemia. 2023 Mar 8. In: StatPearls [Internet]. Treasure Island (FL): StatPearls Publishing; 2025. PMID: 33620846.
23. van der Lugt NM, Smits-Wintjens VE, van Zwieten PH, Walther FJ. Short and long term outcome of neonatal hyperglycemia in very preterm infants: a retrospective follow-up study. BMC Pediatr. 2010;10:52.
24. Butorac Ahel I, Lah Tomulić K, Vlašić Cicvarić I, Žuvić M, Baraba Dekanić K, Šegulja S, Bilić Čače I. Incidence and risk factors for glucose disturbances in premature infants. Medicina (Kaunas). 2022;58:1295.

25. Capone K, Sriram S, Patton T, Weinstein D, Newton E, Wroblewski K, Sentongo T. Effects of chromium on glucose tolerance in infants receiving parenteral nutrition therapy. Nutr Clin Pract. 2018;33:426–32.
26. Burgess L, Morgan C, Mayes K, Tan M. Plasma arginine levels and blood glucose control in very preterm infants receiving 2 different parenteral nutrition regimens. JPEN J Parenter Enteral Nutr. 2014;38:243–53.
27. Gruenwald P, Minh HN. Evaluation of body and organ weights in perinatal pathology. I. Normal standards derived from autopsies. Am J Cin Pathol. 1960;34:247–53.
28. Shelley HJ. Glycogen reserves and their changes at birth and in anoxia. Br Med Bull. 1961;17:137–43.
29. Widdowson EM, Spray CM. Chemical development in utero. Arch Dis Child. 1951;26:205–14.
30. Ziegler EE, O'Donnell AM, Nelson SE, Fomon SJ. Body composition of the reference fetus. Growth. 1976;40:329–41.
31. Harris A, Naylor RN. Pediatric monogenic diabetes: a unique challenge and opportunity. Pediatr Ann. 2019;48:e319–25.
32. Uthaya S, Modi N. Practical preterm parenteral nutrition: systematic literature review and recommendations for practice. Early Hum Dev. 2014;90:747–53.
33. Hay WW Jr. Neonatal hyper- and hypoglycemia: why are they still controversial? Neonatology. 2011;100:336–7.
34. Vasu V, Thomas EL, Durighel G, Hyde MJ, Bell JD, Modi N. Early nutritional determinants of intrahepatocellular lipid deposition in preterm infants at term age. Int J Obes (Lond). 2013;37:500–4.
35. Leos RA, Anderson MJ, Chen X, Pugmire J, Anderson KA, Limesand SW. Chronic exposure to elevated norepinephrine suppresses insulin secretion in fetal sheep with placental insufficiency and intrauterine growth restriction. Am J Physiol Endocrinol Metab. 2010;298:E770–8.
36. Chen X, Kelly AC, Yates DT, Macko AR, Lynch RM, Limesand SW. Islet adaptations in fetal sheep persist following chronic exposure to high norepinephrine. J Endocrinol. 2017;232:285–95.
37. Valverde E, Pellicer A, Madero R, Elorza D, Quero J, Cabañas F. Dopamine versus epinephrine for cardiovascular support in low birth weight infants: analysis of systemic effects and neonatal clinical outcomes. Pediatrics. 2006;117:e1213–22.
38. Louik C, Mitchell AA, Epstein MF, Shapiro S. Risk factors for neonatal hyperglycemia associated with 10% dextrose infusion. Am J Dis Child. 1985;139:783–6.
39. Phadke D, Beller JP, Tribble C. The disparate effects of epinephrine and norepinephrine on hyperglycemia in cardiovascular surgery. Heart Surg Forum. 2018;21:E522–6.
40. Wesolowski SR, Hay WW Jr. Role of placental insufficiency and intrauterine growth restriction on the activation of fetal hepatic glucose production. Mol Cell Endocrinol. 2016;435:61–8.
41. Thorn SR, Brown LD, Rozance PJ, Hay WW Jr, Friedman JE. Increased hepatic glucose production in fetal sheep with intrauterine growth restriction is not suppressed by insulin. Diabetes. 2013;62:65–73.
42. Zarlengo KM, Battaglia FC, Fennessey P, Hay WW Jr. Relationship between glucose utilization rate and glucose concentration in preterm infants. Biol Neonate. 1986;49:181–9.
43. Dickson JL, Hewett JN, Gunn CA, Lynn A, Shaw GM, Chase JG. On the problem of patient-specific endogenous glucose production in neonates on stochastic targeted glycemic control. J Diabetes Sci Technol. 2013;7(4):913–27.
44. Chacko SK, Sunehag AL. Gluconeogenesis continues in premature infants receiving total parenteral nutrition. Arch Dis Child Fetal Neonatal Ed. 2010;95:F413–8.
45. van Kempen AAMW, Ackermans MT, Endert E, Kok JH, Sauerwein HP. Glucose production in response to glucagon is comparable in preterm AGA and SGA infants. Clin Nutr. 2005;24:727–36.
46. Van Kempen AA, Romijn JA, Ruiter AF, Ackermans MT, Endert E, Hoekstra JH, Kok JH, Sauerwein HP. Adaptation of glucose production and gluconeogenesis to diminishing glucose infusion in preterm infants at varying gestational ages. Pediatr Res. 2003;53:628–34.

47. Sunehag AL. Parenteral glycerol enhances gluconeogenesis in very premature infants. Pediatr Res. 2003;53:635–41.
48. Girard J. Gluconeogenesis in late fetal and early neonatal life. Biol Neonate. 1986;50:237–58.
49. Rozance PJ, Limesand SW, Barry JS, Brown LD, Hay WW Jr. Glucose replacement to euglycemia causes hypoxia, acidosis, and decreased insulin secretion in fetal sheep with intrauterine growth restriction. Pediatr Res. 2009;5:72–8.
50. Fowden AL. Pancreatic insulin production and carbohydrate metabolism in the fetus. In: Albrecht EG, Pepe GJ, editors. Perinatal endocrinology. Perinatal Press; 1985. p. 78.
51. Ogilvy-Stuart AL, Beardsall K. Management of hyperglycaemia in the preterm infant. Arch Dis Child Fetal Neonatal Ed. 2010;95:F126–31.
52. Dweck HS, Cassady G. Glucose intolerance in infants of very low birth weight. I. Incidence of hyperglycemia in infants of birth weights 1,100 grams or less. Pediatrics. 1974;53:189–95.
53. Zamir I, Stoltz Sjöström E, van den Berg J, Berhan Y, Naumburg E, Domellöf M. Glucose disturbances in very low-birthweight infants-results from the prospective LIGHT study. Acta Paediatr. 2024;113:2556–63.
54. Spear ML, Reeves G, Pearlman SA. Diabetic ketoacidosis after steroid administration for bronchopulmonary dysplasia: a case report. J Perinatol. 1993;13:232–4.
55. Brown LD. Endocrine regulation of fetal skeletal muscle growth: impact on future metabolic health. J Endocrinol. 2014;221:R13–29.
56. Mitanchez-Mokhtari D, Lahlou N, Kieffer F, Magny JF, Roger M, Voyer M. Both relative insulin resistance and defective islet beta-cell processing of proinsulin are responsible for transient hyperglycemia in extremely preterm infants. Pediatrics. 2004;113:537–41.
57. Salis ER, Reith DM, Wheeler BJ, Broadbent RS, Medlicott NJ. Insulin resistance, glucagon-like peptide-1 and factors influencing glucose homeostasis in neonates. Arch Dis Child Fetal Neonatal Ed. 2017;102:F162–6.
58. Stoll B, Horst DA, Cui L, Chang X, Ellis KJ, Hadsell DL, Suryawan A, Kurundkar A, Maheshwari A, Davis TA, Burrin DG. Chronic parenteral nutrition induces hepatic inflammation, steatosis, and insulin resistance in neonatal pigs. J Nutr. 2010;140:2193–200.
59. Raghavan S, Brishti MA, Bernardelli A, Mata-Daboin A, Jaggar JH, Leo MD. Extracellular glucose and dysfunctional insulin receptor signaling independently upregulate arterial smooth muscle TMEM16A expression. Am J Physiol Cell Physiol. 2024;326:C1237–47.
60. Paauw ND, Stegeman R, de Vroede MAMJ, Termote JUM, Freund MW, Breur JMPJ. Neonatal cardiac hypertrophy: the role of hyperinsulinism-a review of literature. Eur J Pediatr. 2020;179:39–50.

Chapter 10
Adverse Effects of Acute and Persistent Neonatal Hyperglycemia

William W. Hay, Jr. and Jane Alsweiler

There are many complications of hyperglycemia in older children and adults, but in many cases, it has been difficult to dissociate such complications specific to hyperglycemia from other problems, such as malnutrition and coincident pathophysiology. Such complications include increased morbidity and mortality, impaired immunity, increased infection rates, poor wound healing, suppressed autophagy, cellular repair, and organ recovery, and loss of skeletal and cardiac muscle. Evidence for such problems in hyperglycemic newborn infants is lacking or uncertain, most likely because no one has looked for it. If we did look, what would we see?

In fact, there are a large number of complications of neonatal hyperglycemia when maximal glucose oxidative capacity (>8–10 mg/kg/min) and deposition in glycogen are exceeded. The most common of these are shown in Tables 10.1, 10.2, and 10.3.

Both IDMs and infants of obese mothers with pre-gestational diabetes have right ventricular dysfunction that persists well beyond resolution of septal hypertrophy [5]. In part this is due to insulin resistance and amplified sympathetic nervous and renin-angiotensin-aldosterone systems [6]. The common link may be accumulation of collagen in the myocardium with fibrosis, likely the result of prolonged hyperglycemia with advanced glycation end products and excessive production of oxygen free radicals [7]. If such maternal hyperglycemia persists, cardiac Akt-related insulin-signaling can be inhibited, attenuating insulin-sensitive cardiac glucose

W. W. Hay, Jr. (✉)
University of Colorado, Denver, CO, USA
e-mail: bill.hay@ucdenver.edu

J. Alsweiler
Department of Paediatrics: Child and Youth Health, School of Medicine,
University of Auckland, Auckland, New Zealand
e-mail: j.alsweiler@auckland.ac.nz

D. H. Adamkin, W. W. Hay, Jr. (eds.), *Disorders of Neonatal Glycemia*,
https://doi.org/10.1007/978-3-032-29094-6_10

Table 10.1 Complications of neonatal hyperglycemia in IDMs

Hyperosmolarity, polyuria, dehydration, acidosis, hyponatremia, and hypokalemia. (these are not as common anymore due to more careful fluid and electrolyte management and limited IV dextrose infusions).
↑ Energy expenditure (glucose-to-fat synthesis is energy expensive)
↑ Oxygen consumption (potentially leading to hypoxia)
↑ Carbon dioxide production (potentially leading to greater tachypnea)

Table 10.2 Complications of neonatal hyperglycemia that are similar to those in infants of diabetic mothers (IDMs), especially when neonatal hyperglycemia is chronic

↑ Fat deposition in excess of lean mass
↑ Inflammatory fatty infiltration of heart and liver
↓ Vascular integrity leading to poor peripheral blood flow and hypertension
↑ Cardiac septal hypertrophy and Right Ventricular dysfunction (most common in IDMs)
↑ Local and systemic inflammatory mediators
↑ Cellular injury from oxidative stress and free radical production in many, likely all, cells including neurons

Table 10.3 Complications of neonatal hyperglycemia

1. Increased risk of mortality among preterm and ELBW/VLBW infants
2. Increased risk of many morbidities among preterm infants. More severe outcomes occur with prolonged but variable hyperglycemia. Neonates with hyperglycemia have an increased risk of the following:
(a) Intracranial hemorrhage (Hyperglycemia may cause intracranial hemorrhage by causing hyperosmolarity with osmotic shifts [2]. Each increment of 18 mg/dL in blood glucose concentration accounts for a rise of 1 mOsm/L in serum osmolarity. If serum osmolarity suddenly exceeds 300 mOsm/L, rapidly shifting water may cause cerebral hemorrhage.
(b) Dehydration due to osmotic diuresis—not common
(c) Electrolyte imbalance occurs due to osmotic diuresis.
(d) Glycosuria can, though rarely does, increase sodium excretion.
(e) Necrotizing enterocolitis [3]
(f) Retinopathy of prematurity [4]
(g) Bronchopulmonary disease
(h) Impaired immunity and increased risk of sepsis
(i) Poor wound healing
(j) Long term impact on adverse neurodevelopmental outcome
(k) Insulin resistance and glucose intolerance
(l) Side effects due to the management of hyperglycemia (Insulin infusion, for example, increases the risks of hypokalemia and hypoglycemia)

Adapted from Balasundaram and Dumpa [1]

metabolism [8]. There also is evidence from in vitro studies and murine animal models that excess glucose can inhibit cardiac muscle maturation through nucleotide biosynthesis. This inhibits cardiac myocyte maturation at genetic, structural, metabolic, electrophysiological, and biomechanical levels by promoting nucleotide biosynthesis through the pentose phosphate pathway. Fetal hears in the murine diabetic pregnancy model show cardiomyopathy with increased mitotic activity and decreased maturity [9].

Excess Glucose Produces Reactive Oxygen Species

Frequently underappreciated and undocumented is the adverse influence of excess cellular glucose uptake from hyperglycemia on over production of reactive oxygen species (ROS) leading to local and then systemic inflammation (Fig. 10.1) [10].

Evidence that this occurs in a neonatal animal (piglet) model receiving excess glucose as part of TPN clearly shows increased activation of inflammatory genes in both liver and skeletal muscle with excess production of circulating inflammatory proteins (Fig. 10.2) [11].

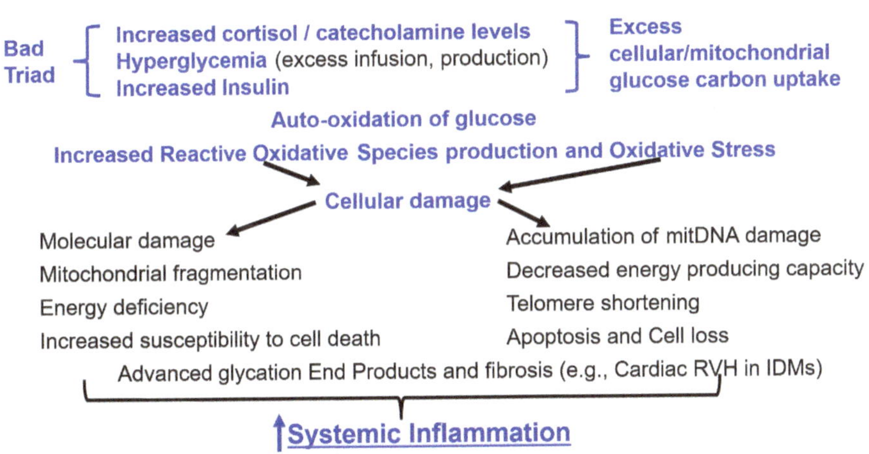

Fig. 10.1 Hyperglycemia in excess of normal oxidation produces damaging free oxygen radicals that lead to local and systemic inflammation. (Adapted from: Picard et al. [10])

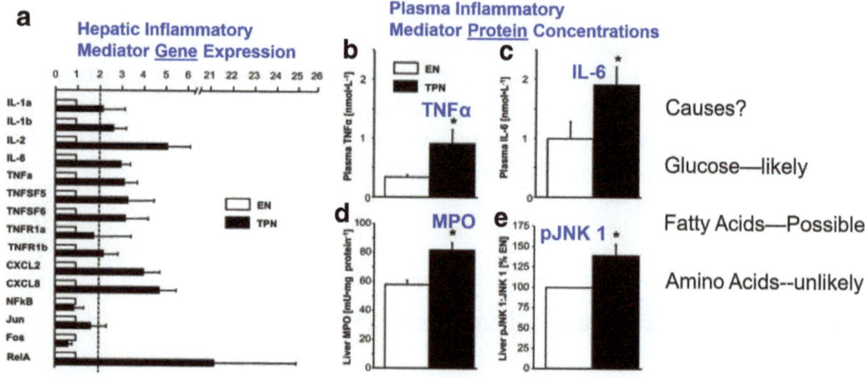

Fig. 10.2 (**a**) Hepatic inflammatory genes, and plasma inflammatory mediator protein concentrations (**b**, TNFα; C, IL-6; D, Myeloperoxidase or MPO; E, pJNK 1) in piglets receiving IV nutrition. (Adapted from: Stoll et al. [11])

Adverse Vascular Effects of Hyperglycemia

Vascular injury, leakage from microvasculature, and related poor wound healing are seldom appreciated in neonates with hyperglycemia but the mechanisms are clear and such problems should be addressed. For example, a study of human aortic endothelial cells (HAECs) and human dermal microvascular (HDMVECs) to observe the functional and proteomic differences potentially contributing to EC heterogeneity found that under high glucose conditions, migration was worsened for both cell types and permeability increased for HDMVECs [12]. Insulin can make such adverse effects worse, as well as adding vascular stiffness that can contribute to hypertension. In a study in rats, for example, hyperglycemia with hyperinsulinemia selectively impaired receptor-dependent, endothelium-dependent relaxation [13]. These studies suggest that hyperglycemia could be a common pathway leading to endothelial dysfunction and abnormal vascular function.

Hyperglycemia Impairs Immunity

Hyperglycemia also impairs leukocyte phagocytic function, decreases complement function, increases pro-inflammatory cytokines, and impairs neutrophil chemotaxis, predisposing hyperglycemic infants to increased susceptibility to infections [14–18]. There even is some data linking hyperglycemia in preterm, VLBW infants who had confirmed SARS-CoV-2 infection and presented with significant hyperglycemia [19].

Also underappreciated is the potential increased risk of sepsis and tissue/organ infection by both bacteria and viruses from hyperglycemia. Bacteria, for example, thrive in the presence of excess glucose, perhaps leading to worse infections and death of the organism. This also might occur in the NICU where bacterial infections are more common as causes of serious sepsis and death [20]. For example, excessively increased blood glucose can compromise GI tract barrier function and promote influx of pathogenic bacteria and their pathological microbial products [21]. Recent data have also shown a causal pathway linking hyperglycemia to an increased risk of microbial gut translocation in both animal models and adult studies [22]. Animal studies in rats also have shown enhanced enteric and diarrheal disease in the presence of hyperglycemia, and in human populations, hyperglycemia, is an independent risk factor for diarrhea incidence and severity during a community *E. coli* outbreak [23]. Persistent hyperglycemia has been associated with NEC, OR 9.49 (95% CI 1.52–59.3) and infection, OR 3.79 (1.40–10.20), which are two major causes of mortality and morbidity for preterm infants) [24]. Hyperglycemia also increases sepsis with mortality in extremely low birthweight infants [3].

For viruses, most believe that they do the opposite; they do not thrive in high glucose conditions. Thus, if an infant has a proven virus infection, perhaps glucose supply might not be as bad. In reality, however, too much glucose also can make viral infections worse by promoting inflammatory cytokines that are specific to the virus and its target organ. For example, excess glucose in the presence of hyperglycemia and influenza virus infection can promote production of inflammatory cytokines in more susceptible pulmonary cells leading to increased lung injury and pneumonia [25].

Hyperglycemia and Mortality and Morbidity

A systematic review and meta-analysis assessed the association between hyperglycemia in preterm neonates (<32 weeks or <1500 g) and mortality and morbidities. Forty-six studies (30 cohort and 16 case control) with data from 34,527 infants were evaluated. Meta-analysis of unadjusted ORs from cohort studies most importantly found that hyperglycemia was significantly associated with mortality, any-grade intraventricular hemorrhage (IVH), severe IVH, any-stage retinopathy of prematurity (ROP), severe ROP, sepsis, chronic lung disease and disability. However, pooling of adjusted ORs found significant associations only for mortality, 'any grade IVH', and 'any stage ROP' [26].

Hyperglycemia and Intraventricular Hemorrhage (IVH)

Long duration of hyperglycemia in the first 96 h of life is particularly associated with severe IVH in preterm infants [26]. Meta-regression analysis has found glucose levels >10 mmol/L to be especially associated with increased odds of mortality compared with <10 mmol/L. Pooled analysis from case-control studies were similar to cohort studies for most outcomes but limited by small sample size. Longer duration of hyperglycemia in particular was associated with adverse outcomes. Hyperglycemia in very preterm infants clearly is associated with higher odds of mortality, any-grade IVH, and any-stage ROP [27].

Hyperglycemia and Retinopathy of Prematurity (ROP)

There are several recent studies that have assessed the specific association of hyperglycemia with an increased incidence of retinopathy of prematurity (ROP), even though other studies have not been consistent or conclusive in this regard [28–31]. A comparative analysis of ROP Incidence, IVH incidence, and mortality rates between long-term and short-term hyperglycemia groups showed that there were no statistically significant differences in IVH incidence or mortality rates between the two groups ($p = 0.307$ and $p = 0.134$). However, preterm neonates with prolonged hyperglycemia duration showed a significantly higher incidence of retinopathy of prematurity (ROP) ($p = 0.007$) [32] A more recent study, however, showed a greater number of infants with ROP who had early (days 1–7) sustained glucose concentrations >100 mg/dL [33]. Another study confirmed that there is an independent association between the occurrence of hyperglycemic events during first postnatal week and later development of ROP requiring treatment, when adjusted for other known risk factors [34].

But isn't this the same period of retinal oxygen toxicity? It is indeed true that higher glucose concentrations are associated with the development of severe ROP, during days 2–5 with hyperoxia [35], but this association also occurs during the following days, 5–16, without hyperoxic conditions and thus likely independent of hyperoxia [4, 36]. Hyperglycemia induced increased insulin production might make this worse by promoting increased retinal cell glucose uptake, glucose oxidation, and ROS production. Interestingly, amino acids might limit this by promoting IGF-1 production [37] that may be protective against ROP [38]. Animal models in general support the adverse effect of hyperglycemia on ROP development. In mice, for example, modeling hyperglycemia-associated Phase I ROP, showed significant changes in retinal amino acids (including most decreased L-leucine, L-isoleucine, and L-valine) [39].

Hyperglycemia Adversely Affects Neuronal Development

Hyperglycemia increases central nervous system permeability, oxidative stress, and leads to microglia activation and astrocytosis, as well as regulation of DNA repair mechanisms, compromising neuronal and glial cell integrity [40]. This can lead to long-term changes in synaptogenesis and behavior [41]. In a study in neonatal rats, brain weight was reduced and apoptosis, tissue malondialdehyde, xanthine oxidase levels, and total oxidant status were significantly increased, whereas total antioxidant status was significantly decreased [42].

Hyperglycemia Worsens Hypoxic Ischemic Encephalopathy (HIE)

Hyperglycemia also appears to be particularly injurious to infants with hypoxic-ischemic encephalopathy (HIE), especially in those infants who receive hypothermia therapy [43]. In one study, for example, 100% of infants who received hypothermia therapy with blood glucose levels >200 mg/dL during the first 24 h of age died or had moderate/severe disability, compared with 54.5% of those with blood glucose <200 mg/dL in this group (p = 0.03). A similar effect was not present in the No-TH group. Hyperglycemia on the first day, therefore, portends poor outcome in newborn infants undergoing TH for HIE [44].

In another study, at every point in the first 12 h after an episode of HIE, hyperglycemia produced more unfavorable outcomes than did hypoglycemia [45]. Furthermore, the odds of predominant watershed/focal-multifocal Infarct injury and basal ganglia and global Injury are highest with hyperglycemia, next-highest with labile (mostly high) values, and least-highest with hypoglycemia, compared with infants with normal blood glucose values during the post-rewarming period after brain and body cooling for HIE [46]. Dysglycemia (hypo-, hyper-, and labile) affects nearly two-thirds of newborns with neonatal encephalopathy and is independently associated with a higher risk of mortality and/or brain lesions on MRI. Adverse outcomes are significantly greater for the group with hyperglycemia (aOR 1.81; 95% CI 1.06–3.11) [47]. In another study of infants with HIE and both hypo- and hyperglycemia, although hypoglycemia occurred at similar rates in severe and moderate HIE (21.4% vs 19.5%; P = 0.67), hyperglycemia was more common in severe HIE (42.3% vs 16.9%; P < 0.001). Compared with euglycemic neonates, both, hypo- and hyperglycemic neonates had an increased aOR (95% confidence interval) for death or NDI (2.62; 1.47–4.67 and 1.77; 1.03–3.03) compared to those with euglycemia. Hypoglycemic neonates had an increased aOR for both death (2.85; 1.09–7.43) and NDI (2.50; 1.09–7.43), whereas hyperglycemic neonates had increased aOR of 2.52 (1.10–5.77) for death, but not NDI [48, 49]. Higher blood glucose concentrations also are associated with worse motor outcomes and death ("Poor Outcomes") in asphyxiated term infants [50, 51]. Similar results showing worse HIE outcomes in infants with hyperglycemia and HIE than those with hypoglycemia and HIE were documented using continuous glucose monitoring (CGM) [52].

In yet another study of infants with HIE and simultaneous measurement of glucose concentrations in the circulation and aEEG recordings, compared with epochs of normoglycemia, epochs of hyperglycemia were associated with worse aEEG background scores (B 1.120, 95% CI 0.501–1.738, P < 0.001), less sleep–wake cycling (B 0.587, 95% CI 0.417–0.757, P < 0.001) and more electrographic seizures (B 0.433, 95% CI 0.185–0.681, P = 0.001), after adjusting for hypoxia–ischemia severity. In neonates with encephalopathy, epochs of hyperglycemia are temporally associated with worse global brain function and seizures, even after adjusting for hypoxia–ischemia severity [53]. Whether hyperglycemia causes neuronal injury or is simply a marker of severe brain injury requires further study [54].

Increased blood glucose concentrations also can promote the release of proinflammatory cytokines, which have been shown to lower seizure thresholds and increase neuronal excitability [55]. An imbalance of the excitatory neurotransmitter glutamate can result from hyperglycemia. Because of this imbalance, there may be excessive neuronal activation, which raises the risk of seizures [56]. Variations in glucose levels can affect how well ion channels function in neurons, which can upset the electrolyte balance. These alterations can cause neuronal hyperexcitability and seizures [57]. Clearly, hyperglycemia independently can worsen several adverse outcomes of HIE [58].

Hyperglycemia with Parenteral Nutrition and Adverse Neurodevelopment

Neonatal hyperglycemia related to parenteral nutrition also adversely affects long-term (2 years) neurodevelopment in preterm newborns. The fraction of children with neuro-developmental delays, regardless of condition, is much greater in the presence of hyperglycemia than in normoglycemic control children (Fig. 10.3) [59].

A study from Sweden also showed that early and prolonged hyperglycemia in very preterm infants is associated with reduced brain white matter volume at 2.5 Years [60].

- White matter volume was reduced by 2.4 mL for hyperglycemia days 0–2, p = 0.02.

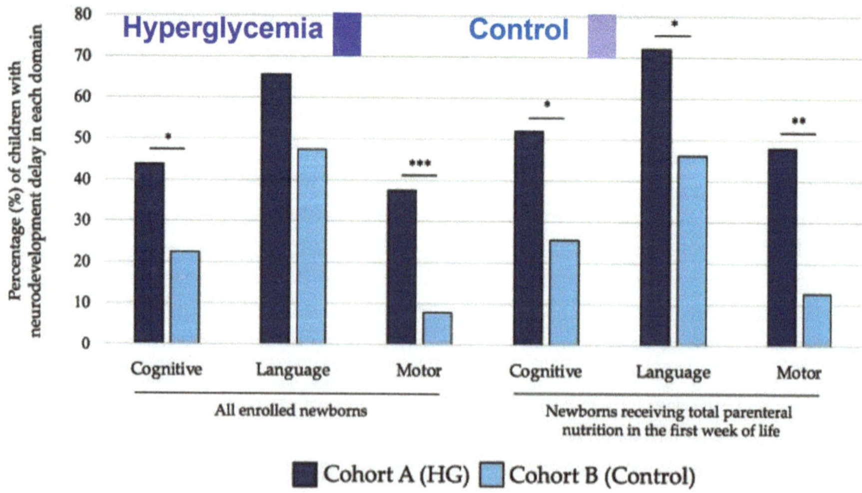

Fig. 10.3 Two-year neurodevelopmental delays in hyperglycemic vs. normoglycemic preterm neonates. (From: Boscarino et al. [59])

- White matter volume was reduced by 16.5 mL for prolonged (>2 days) hyperglycemia >8.3 mmol/L (>150 mg/dL), p = 0.042
- Total brain volume was reduced by 27.2 mL for prolonged (>2 days) hyperglycemia >8.3 mmol/L (>150 mg/dL), p = 0.051 and with worse cognitive and motor outcomes at 2.5 years
- Bayley-III Cognitive Score was reduced by 1.14 points (p = 0.032) and Bayley-III motor score by 1.75 points (P = 0.027) for hyperglycemia days 0–2.
- Bayley-III Motor Score was reduced by 4.7 points for prolonged (>2 days) hyperglycemia >10 mmol/L (>180 mg/dL), P = 0.014.

Similar observations haven been noted among preterm infants with hyperglycemia early after birth during the first week of life, but particularly during the first 24 h of life when brain MRI abnormalities at term-equivalent age in extremely preterm infants have reduced white matter and increased risk for death [29].

Duration of Hyperglycemia

And another study showed that longer duration of hyperglycemia is associated with worse cognitive and motor developmental outcomes at 6.5 years. In this study, of 533 preterm infants born <27 gestational weeks during 2004–2007; 436 survivors were assessed at 6.5 years. For longer durations of neonatal hyperglycemia >8 mmol/L, for each day with hyperglycemia there was a decrease of 0.33 points (95% CI 0.03 to 0.62) in Full Scale IQ. Neonatal hyperglycemia >8 mmol/L (>144 mg/dL) occurring on 3 consecutive days was associated with lower MABC-2 scores (Movement Assessment Battery for Children—adjusted mean difference: −4.90; 95% CI −8.90 to −0.89). For each day with hyperglycemia >8 mmol/L (>144 mg/dL), there was a decrease of 0.55 points in MABC-2 total score (95% CI 0.17 to 0.93). Importantly, insulin treatment was not associated with any of the outcome measure, which is not surprising, as circulating insulin does not promote glucose uptake by the brain—excess glucose is the problem, not insulin. This developmental study clearly shows that prolonged neonatal hyperglycemia >8 mmol/L (>144 mg/dL) is associated with lower intelligence scores and worse motor outcomes at 2.5 and 6.5 years [61].

Hyperglycemia and Increased Risk of Death

Most disturbingly, an important study showed that early enhanced parenteral nutrition with prolonged hyperglycemia was associated with increased risk of death among EPT/VPT, extremely low-birth-weight infants [62]. In this study, early enhanced parenteral nutrition itself was not predictive of mortality, but severe hyperglycemia was predictive of mortality, independent of risk factors except gestational age at birth and early postnatal clinical risk index. In a study of 252 preterm infants with low gestational age (<27 weeks), elevated median blood glucose levels, and/or repeatedly elevated blood glucose levels ≥150 mg/dL were associated with significantly increased mortality [63].

Other studies also have documented increased risk of death as well as other morbidities in preterm infants with both acute and prolonged hyperglycemia [3, 25, 29, 64]. Mortality also is much higher in preterm baboons, even if in these animals there are no associated short-term morbidities, adding evidence that hyperglycemia is causal even for mortality [65, 66]. A primary cause of mortality and severe morbidity with hyperglycemia is its association with intraventricular and intracerebral hemorrhage. In one study of preterm infants admitted to NICU, severe IVH was significantly associated with isolated hyperglycemia (adjusted relative risk [aRR], 2.46; 95% CI, 1.16, 5.23), even though both hypo- and hyperglycemia were associated with mortality [67].

Hyperglycemia, Illness, Nutrition

It also is important to note that hyperglycemia is not simply a marker of illness and poor nutrition. Causality for increased morbidity and mortality was convincingly demonstrated in preterm lambs that were infused with dextrose to produce hyperglycemia (10.8 ± 0.6 mmol/L) for 12 days vs. a saline-infused control group (5.6 ± 0.1 mmol/L). The dextrose infused hyperglycemic preterm lambs had increased morbidity, particularly fever, but also leg shortening, and increased mortality. Insulin infusion producing control level glucose concentrations over the same period in a third group of preterm lambs attenuated the increased mortality and morbidity, but not the reduced growth, indicating that perhaps the hyperglycemia and insulin treatment did not normalize amino acid utilization for protein synthesis [68]. Another study in preterm infants showed that longer duration of hyperglycemia and worse neurodevelopmental outcomes were independent of increasing severity of illness and worse nutrition. There was no change in Bayley cognition, language, or motor scores despite increasing protein and energy deficits [69]. Mechanisms for neuronal injury remain insufficiently studied. However, it is known that hyperglycemia reduces antioxidant superoxide dismutase (SOD) activity and glutathione (GSH), a potent antioxidant and detoxifying agent, and increases oxidative stress (lipid peroxidation and total thiol levels). Hyperglycemia also inhibits retinoic acid–induced neuronal differentiation [70]. In a rat pup model with 11 days (thus, relatively chronic) of subcutaneous dextrose injection, neuronal density in the dentate gyrus and the parietal cortex were progressively reduced, while oxidant status progressively increased and antioxidant status decreased [43]. There also is evidence that astrocyte-endothelial signal transduction exposure to high glucose causes overproduction of VEGF and abnormal proliferation of endothelial cells, loss of gap junction connexin 43 (Cx43, which plays an important role in autocrine and paracrine signaling interactions that mediate gliovascular cross talk through secreted products), expression, cell membrane gap junctions, and astrocyte function, which correlate with the impairment in blood-brain barrier [71].

Hyperglycemia and Growth Restriction

Even growth may be reduced with prolonged hyperglycemia in very low birth weight preterm infants, though linear growth reduction might be compensated by reduced adiposity. Downregulation of the growth hormone axis may be responsible. These changes could influence long-term growth and cognitive development, adding to the short term adverse effects of hyperglycemia in preterm infants on essentially every cell and organ in the infant's body [72, 73]. Furthermore, animal data from experimental studies have shown that neonatal hyperglycemia in preterm lambs causes increased mortality and morbidity and decreases growth. Insulin treatment to restore euglycemia attenuated the increased mortality and morbidity, but not the decreased growth, indicating that hyperglycemia is causal for reduced growth in early development [68].

Hyperglycemia and Renal Injury

Chronic hyperglycemia in adults with diabetes causes renal damage, but it also is the case that acute hyperglycemia can damage renal tubules. Many preterm infants suffer renal damage associated with hypoxic-ischemic insults, an increasingly recognized and relatively common problem. Since such conditions are also associated with acute hyperglycemia, it is reasonable to consider that hypoxic-ischemic renal injury might be aggravated by simultaneous hyperglycemia. In one study it was noted that acute hyperglycemia causes renal tubular morphological and functional injuries in a dose-dependent manner. Acute hyperglycemia could inhibit mitophagy through AMPK/mTOR pathway, which would aggravate mitochondria damage and renal tubular impairment [74].

Longer Term Adverse Outcomes of Neonatal Hyperglycemia

While associations between neonatal hyperglycemia and adverse short-term outcomes, including mortality, retinopathy of prematurity, and intraventricular haemorrhage, have been described [26], high-quality data on its long-term metabolic, cardiovascular and neurodevelopmental consequences remain limited. Concerns persist that early hyperglycemia may contribute to both neurodevelopmental delays and later metabolic dysfunction. It is well established that preterm infants are at increased risk of developing type 2 diabetes in adulthood [75, 76]. However, the specific neonatal factors driving impaired glucose regulation in later life, including the potential role of hyperglycemia, are not yet clearly defined.

Animal studies allow us to generate knowledge of potential long-term complications. Newborn rats made hyperglycaemic have significant changes in pancreatic development [77]. Lambs born preterm had later reduced beta-cell mass, altered insulin secretion, and altered pancreatic mRNA expression compared with lambs born at term [78]. In addition to the effects of preterm birth, hyperglycemia induced by dextrose overload in the neonatal period increased beta-cell apoptosis, further exacerbating some of the effects of preterm birth on pancreatic mRNA expression. If the same is true in humans, then babies born extremely preterm who experience neonatal hyperglycemia may be at greater risk of type 2 diabetes in later life. To date the only evidence from human studies is from preterm babies randomized to tight glycaemic control with insulin. These infants had lower fasting glucose concentrations compared to babies randomized to standard care but did not have any difference in glucose tolerance at 7 years of age [65].

Insulin treatment for neonatal hyperglycemia has been associated with the development of cardiac hypertrophy [79]. Tight glycaemic control with insulin for treatment of neonatal hyperglycemia did not affect the development of ventricular hypertrophy in the neonatal period compared to babies who received standard care with insulin [80]. However, children who as preterm babies had neonatal hyperglycaemia had higher systolic and diastolic blood pressure [81], a higher-than-expected incidence of hypertension [65], and thicker intraventricular septal wall and left ventricular posterior wall thickness at 6–7 years of age [82]. These findings raise the possibility that neonatal hyperglycemia may increase the risk of cardiometabolic disease in later life.

From a neurodevelopmental perspective, hyperglycemic newborn rat pups treated with intranasal insulin, which bypasses the blood brain barrier, had improved long-term hippocampal development [83]. In preterm babies several systematic reviews of the evidence of longer-term neurodevelopmental outcomes following neonatal hyperglycemia found 6–8 studies, mostly observational, with low quality evidence [28, 84]. For example, a retrospective follow-up study at 2 years of age was conducted among 859 infants ≤32 weeks of gestation admitted to a tertiary neonatal center between January 2002 and December 2006. Thirty-three survivors treated with insulin for hyperglycemia and 63 matched controls without hyperglycemia were evaluated at a corrected age of 2 years. Outcome measures consisted of growth (weight, length, and head circumference) and neurological and behavioral development. Mortality was higher in very preterm infants with hyperglycemia treated with insulin during the neonatal period ($p < 0.001$). At 2 years of age survivors showed normal growth, but a higher incidence of neurological ($p < 0.035$) and behavioral ($p < 0.021$) problems [85]. Meta-analyses, which might have guided interpretation of the existing findings from such limited studies, have not been sufficiently conducted because of the clinical and methodological heterogeneity in the small number of published studies.

Conclusions

Neonatal hyperglycemia is common, compounded by many conditions starting in the fetus and developing after birth that increase the risk of hyperglycemia and its complications, it gets worse the longer it persists, and it is pathological, perhaps even lethal. Specifically for preterm infants, preterm birth is associated with long-term risks of impaired glucose regulation and adverse neurodevelopmental outcomes. While neonatal hyperglycemia is linked to short-term morbidity and mortality, its impact on later insulin sensitivity, cardiovascular health and brain development remains unclear. Animal studies suggest that hyperglycemia may exacerbate pancreatic dysfunction, and human trials have shown only limited neurodevelopmental benefit if any from tight glycemic control despite increased hyperglycemia risk. High-quality longitudinal studies are needed to clarify whether neonatal hyperglycemia contributes to adverse metabolic and neurodevelopmental outcomes, and whether it represents a modifiable risk factor. Finding better strategies to manage hyperglycemia may improve outcome of very preterm infants.

References

1. Balasundaram P, Dumpa V. Neonatal hyperglycemia. 2023 Mar 8. In: StatPearls [Internet]. Treasure Island (FL): StatPearls Publishing; 2025. PMID: 33620846.
2. Pildes RS. Neonatal hyperglycemia. J Pediatr. 1986;109:905–7.
3. Kao LS, Morris BH, Lally KP, Stewart CD, Huseby V, Kennedy KA. Hyperglycemia and morbidity and mortality in extremely low birth weight infants. J Perinatol. 2006;26:730–6.
4. Garg R, Agthe AG, Donohue PK, Lehmann CU. Hyperglycemia and retinopathy of prematurity in very low birth weight infants. J Perinatol. 2003;23:186–94.
5. Cade WT, Levy PT, Tinius RA, Patel MD, Choudhry S, Holland MR, Singh GK, Cahill AG. Markers of maternal and infant metabolism are associated with ventricular dysfunction in infants of obese women with type 2 diabetes. Pediatr Res. 2017;82:768–75.
6. Tadic M, Ivanovic B, Cuspidi C. Metabolic syndrome and right ventricle: an updated review. Eur J Intern Med. 2013;24:608–16.
7. Rösen P, Du X, Tschöpe D. Role of oxygen derived radicals for vascular dysfunction in the diabetic heart: prevention by alpha-tocopherol? Mol Cell Biochem. 1998;188:103–11.
8. Kawaharada R, Masuda H, Chen Z, Blough E, Kohama T, Nakamura A. Intrauterine hyperglycemia-induced inflammatory signaling via the receptor for advanced glycation end products in the cardiac muscle of the infants of diabetic mother rats. Eur J Nutr. 2018;57:2701–12.
9. Nakano H, Minami I, Braas D, Pappoe H, Wu X, Sagadevan A, Vergnes L, Fu K, Morselli M, Dunham C, Ding X, Stieg AZ, Gimzewski JK, Pellegrini M, Clark PM, Reue K, Lusis AJ, Ribalet B, Kurdistani SK, Christofk H, Nakatsuji N, Nakano A. Glucose inhibits cardiac muscle maturation through nucleotide biosynthesis. elife. 2017;6:e29330.
10. Picard M, Juster RP, McEwen BS. Mitochondrial allostatic load puts the 'gluc' back in glucocorticoids. Nat Rev Endocrinol. 2014;10:303–31.
11. Stoll B, Horst DA, Cui L, Chang X, Ellis KJ, Hadsell DL, Suryawan A, Kurundkar A, Maheshwari A, Davis TA, Burrin DG. Chronic parenteral nutrition induces hepatic inflammation, steatosis, and insulin resistance in neonatal pigs. J Nutr. 2010;140:2193–200.

12. Minjares M, Jaiswal R, Li H, Zhang X, Shvartsman S, Yi Z, Wang JM. Proteomic and functional analysis on endothelial cell heterogeneity identifies key regulators in hyperglycemia-induced dysfunction. Am J Physiol Cell Physiol. 2025;329:C1894–906.
13. Pieper GM, Meier DA, Hager SR. Endothelial dysfunction in a model of hyperglycemia and hyperinsulinemia. Am J Phys Heart Circ Phys. 1995;269:H845–50.
14. Marik PE, Raghavan M. Stress-hyperglycemia, insulin and immunomodulation in sepsis. Intensive Care Med. 2004;30:748–56.
15. Nielson CP, Hindson DA. Inhibition of polymorphonuclear leukocyte respiratory burst by elevated glucose concentrations in vitro. Diabetes. 1989;38:1031–5.
16. Vanhorebeek I, De Vos R, Mesotten D, Wouters PJ, De Wolf-Peeters C, Van den Berghe G. Protection of hepatocyte mitochondrial ultrastructure and function by strict blood glucose control with insulin in critically ill patients. Lancet. 2005;365:53–9.
17. Turina M, Fry DE, Polk HC Jr. Acute hyperglycemia and the innate immune system: clinical, cellular, and molecular aspects. Crit Care Med. 2005;33:1624–33.
18. Angelika D, Etika R, Utomo MT, Ladydi L, Sampurna MTA, Handayani KD, Ugrasena IDG, Sauer PJ. The incidence of and risk factors for hyperglycemia and hypoglycemia in preterm infants receiving early-aggressive parenteral nutrition. Heliyon. 2023;9:e18966.
19. Boly TJ, Reyes-Hernandez ME, Daniels EC, Kibbi N, Bermick JR, Elgin TG. Hyperglycemia and cytopenias as signs of SARS-CoV-2 delta variant infection in preterm infants. Pediatrics. 2022;149:e2021055331.
20. Wang A, Huen SC, Luan HH, Yu S, Zhang C, Gallezot JD, Booth CJ, Medzhitov R. Opposing effects of fasting metabolism on tissue tolerance in bacterial and viral inflammation. Cell. 2016;166:1512–25.
21. Anhê FF, Barra NG, Schertzer JD. Glucose alters the symbiotic relationships between gut microbiota and host physiology. Am J Physiol Endocrinol Metab. 2020;318:E111–6.
22. Thaiss CA, Levy M, Grosheva I, Zheng D, Soffer E, Blacher E, Braverman S, Tengeler AC, Barak O, Elazar M, Ben-Zeev R, Lehavi-Regev D, Katz MN, Pevsner-Fischer M, Gertler A, Halpern Z, Harmelin A, Aamar S, Serradas P, Grosfeld A, Shapiro H, Geiger B, Elinav E. Hyperglycemia drives intestinal barrier dysfunction and risk for enteric infection. Science. 2018;359:1376–83.
23. Bhatwa A, Lau TC, McPhee JB, Anhê FF, Anhê GF, Fang H, Barra NG, Li Y, Duggan BM, Chan DY, Gunn E, Gagnon C, Tchernof A, Marette A, Morrison KM, Coombes BK, Schertzer JD. Hyperglycemia worsens gut bacterial infection through intestinal Wnt, but independent of endotoxemia or obesity. Am J Physiol Endocrinol Metab. 2025;329:E441–54.
24. Beardsall K, Vanhaesebrouck S, Ogilvy-Stuart AL, Vanhole C, Palmer CR, Ong K, vanWeissenbruch M, Midgley P, Thompson M, Thio M, Cornette L, Ossuetta I, Iglesias I, Theyskens C, de Jong M, Gill B, Ahluwalia JS, de Zegher F, Dunger DB. Prevalence and determinants of hyperglycemia in very low birth weight infants: cohort analyses of the NIRTURE study. J Pediatr. 2010;15:715–719.e1–3.
25. Wang Q, Fang P, He R, Li M, Yu H, Zhou L, Yi Y, Wang F, Rong Y, Zhang Y, Chen A, Peng N, Lin Y, Lu M, Zhu Y, Peng G, Rao L, Liu S. *O*-GlcNAc transferase promotes influenza A virus-induced cytokine storm by targeting interferon regulatory factor-5. Sci Adv. 2020;6:eaaz7086.
26. Rath CP, Shivamallappa M, Muthusamy S, Rao SC, Patole S. Outcomes of very preterm infants with neonatal hyperglycaemia: a systematic review and meta-analysis. Arch Dis Child Fetal Neonatal Ed. 2022;107:269–80.
27. Auerbach A, Eventov-Friedman S, Arad I, Peleg O, Bdolah-Abram T, Bar-Oz B, Zangen DH. Long duration of hyperglycemia in the first 96 hours of life is associated with severe intraventricular hemorrhage in preterm infants. J Pediatr. 2013;163:388–93.
28. Paulsen ME, Brown SJ, Satrom KM, Scheurer JM, Ramel SE, Rao RB. Long-term outcomes after early neonatal hyperglycemia in VLBW infants: a systematic review. Neonatology. 2021;118:509–21.
29. Alexandrou G, Skiöld B, Karlén J, Tessma MK, Norman M, Adén U, Vanpée M. Early hyperglycemia is a risk factor for death and white matter reduction in preterm infants. Pediatrics. 2010;125:e584–91.

30. Lei C, Duan J, Ge G, Zhang M. Association between neonatal hyperglycemia and retinopathy of prematurity: a meta-analysis. Eur J Pediatr. 2021;180:3433–42.
31. Au SCL, Tang S-M, Rong S-S, Chen L-J, Yam JCS. Association between hyperglycemia and retinopathy of prematurity: a systemic review and meta-analysis. Sci Rep. 2015;5:9091.
32. Leung M, Black J, Bloomfield FH, Gamble GD, Harding JE, Jiang Y, Poppe T, Thompson B, Tottman AC, Wouldes TA, Alsweiler JM, PIANO Study Group. Effects of neonatal hyperglycemia on retinopathy of prematurity and visual outcomes at 7 years of age: a matched cohort study. J Pediatr. 2020;223:42–50.e2.
33. Zhu J, He X, Guo M. Association of early hyperglycemia with morbidity and mortality in very low birth weight infants. BMC Pediatr. 2025;25:667.
34. Mohsen L, Abou-Alam M, El-Dib M, Labib M, Elsada M, Aly H. A prospective study on hyperglycemia and retinopathy of prematurity. J Perinatol. 2014;34:453–7.
35. Slidsborg C, Jensen LB, Rasmussen SC, Fledelius HC, Greisen G, Cour M. Early postnatal hyperglycaemia is a risk factor for treatment-demanding retinopathy of prematurity. Br J Ophthalmol. 2018;102:14–8.
36. Esmail J, Sakaria RP, Dhanireddy R. Early hyperglycemia is associated with increased incidence of severe retinopathy of prematurity in extremely low birth weight infants. Am J Perinatol. 2024;41:e2842–9.
37. Chavez-Valdez R, McGowan J, Cannon E, Lehmann CU. Contribution of early glycemic status in the development of severe retinopathy of prematurity in a cohort of ELBW infants. J Perinatol. 2011;31:749–56.
38. Cakir B, Hellström W, Tomita Y, Fu Z, Liegl R, Winberg A, Hansen-Pupp I, Ley D, Hellström A, Löfqvist C, Smith LE. IGF1, serum glucose, and retinopathy of prematurity in extremely preterm infants. JCI Insight. 2020;2(5):e140363.
39. Fang JL, Sorita A, Carey WA, Colby CE, Murad MH, Alahdab F. Interventions to prevent retinopathy of prematurity: a meta-analysis. Pediatrics. 2016;137:e20153387.
40. Harman JC, Pivodic A, Nilsson AK, Boeck M, Yagi H, Neilsen K, Ko M, Yang J, Kinter M, Hellström A, Fu Z. Postnatal hyperglycemia alters amino acid profile in retinas (model of Phase I ROP). iScience. 2023;26:108021.
41. Sonneville R, Vanhorebeek I, den Hertog HM, Chrétien F, Annane D, Sharshar T, Van den Berghe G. Critical illness-induced dysglycemia and the brain. Intensive Care Med. 2015;41:192–202.
42. Satrom KM, Ennis K, Sweis BM, Matveeva TM, Chen J, Hanson L, Maheshwari A, Rao R. Neonatal hyperglycemia induces CXCL10/CXCR3 signaling and microglial activation and impairs long-term synaptogenesis in the hippocampus and alters behavior in rats. J Neuroinflammation. 2018;15:82.
43. Tayman C, Yis U, Hirfanoglu I, Oztekin O, Göktaş G, Bilgin BC. Effects of hyperglycemia on the developing brain in newborns. Pediatr Neurol. 2014;51:239–45.
44. Efron D, South M, Volpe JJ, Inder T. Cerebral injury in association with profound iatrogenic hyperglycemia in a neonate. Eur J Paediatr Neurol. 2003;7:167–71.
45. Chouthai NS, Sobczak H, Khan R, Subramanian D, Raman S, Rao R. Hyperglycemia is associated with poor outcome in newborn infants undergoing therapeutic hypothermia for hypoxic ischemic encephalopathy. J Neonatal Perinatal Med. 2015;8:125–31.
46. Basu SK, Kaiser JR, Guffey D, Minard CG, Guillet R, Gunn AJ, CoolCap Study Group. Hypoglycaemia and hyperglycaemia are associated with unfavourable outcome in infants with hypoxic ischaemic encephalopathy: a post hoc analysis of the CoolCap Study. Arch Dis Child Fetal Neonatal Ed. 2016;101:F149–55.
47. Basu SK, Ottolini K, Govindan V, Mashat S, Vezina G, Wang Y, Ridore M, Chang T, Kaiser JR, Massaro AN. Early glycemic profile is associated with brain injury patterns on magnetic resonance imaging in hypoxic ischemic encephalopathy. J Pediatr. 2018;203:137–43.
48. Guellec I, Ancel PY, Beck J, Loron G, Chevallier M, Pierrat V, Kayem G, Vilotitch A, Baud O, Ego A, Debillon T. Glycemia and neonatal encephalopathy: outcomes in the LyTONEPAL (Long-Term Outcome of Neonatal Hypoxic EncePhALopathy in the Era of Neuroprotective Treatment With Hypothermia) cohort. J Pediatr. 2023;257:113350.

49. Mietzsch U, Wood TR, Wu TW, Natarajan N, Glass HC, Gonzalez FF, Mayock DE, Comstock BA, Heagerty PJ, Juul SE, Wu YW, HEAL Study Group. Early glycemic state and outcomes of neonates with hypoxic-ischemic encephalopathy. Pediatrics. 2023;152:e2022060965.
50. Puzone S, Diplomatico M, Caredda E, Maietta A, Miraglia Del Giudice E, Montaldo P. Hypoglycaemia and hyperglycaemia in neonatal encephalopathy: a systematic review and meta-analysis. Arch Dis Child Fetal Neonatal Ed. 2023;109:18–25.
51. Spies EE, Lababidi SL, McBride MC. Early hyperglycemia is associated with poor gross motor outcome in asphyxiated term newborns. Pediatr Neurol. 2014;50:586–90.
52. Montaldo P, Caredda E, Pugliese U, Zanfardino A, Delehaye C, Inserra E, Capozzi L, Chello G, Capristo C, Miraglia Del Giudice E, Iafusco D. Continuous glucose monitoring profile during therapeutic hypothermia in encephalopathic infants with unfavorable outcome. Pediatr Res. 2020;88:218–24.
53. Pinchefsky EF, Hahn CD, Kamino D, Chau V, Brant R, Moore AM, Tam EWY. Hyperglycemia and glucose variability are associated with worse brain function and seizures in neonatal encephalopathy: a prospective cohort study. J Pediatr. 2019;209:23–32.
54. Nair J, Kumar V. Is glucose variability associated with worse brain function and seizures in neonatal encephalopathy? J Perinatol. 2020;40:827–30.
55. Hotz AL, Jamali A, Rieser NN, Niklaus S, Aydin E, Myren-Svelstad S, Lalla L, Jurisch-Yaksi N, Yaksi E, Neuhauss SCF. Loss of glutamate transporter eaat2a leads to aberrant neuronal excitability, recurrent epileptic seizures, and basal hypoactivity. Glia. 2022;70:196–214.
56. Giha HA. Hidden chronic metabolic acidosis of diabetes type 2 (CMAD): clues, causes and consequences. Rev Endocr Metab Disord. 2023;24:735–50.
57. Larsen BR, Stoica A, MacAulay N. Managing brain extracellular K(+) during neuronal activity: the physiological role of the Na(+)/K(+)-ATPase subunit isoforms. Front Physiol. 2016;7:141.
58. Nadeem MD, Memon S, Qureshi K, Farooq U, Memon UA, Aparna F, Kachhadia MP, Shahzeen F, Ali S, Varrassi G, Kumar L, Kumar S, Kumar S, Khatri M. Seizing the connection: exploring the interplay between epilepsy and glycemic control in diabetes management. Cureus. 2023;15:e45606.
59. Boscarino G, Conti MG, Gasparini C, Onestà E, Faccioli F, Dito L, Regoli D, Spalice A, Parisi P, Terrin G. Neonatal hyperglycemia related to parenteral nutrition affects long-term neurodevelopment in preterm newborn: a prospective cohort study. Nutrients. 2021;13:1930.
60. Naseh N, Canto Moreira N, Vaz TF, Gonzalez Tamez K, Ferreira H, Kaul YF, Johansson M, Diderholm B, Ahlsson F, Ågren J, Hellström-Westas L. Early hyperglycemia in very preterm infants is associated with reduced white matter volume and worse cognitive and motor outcomes at 2.5 years. Neonatology. 2022;119:745–52.
61. Zamir I, Stoltz Sjöström E, Ahlsson F, Hansen-Pupp I, Serenius F, Domellöf M. Neonatal hyperglycaemia is associated with worse neurodevelopmental outcomes in extremely preterm infants. Arch Dis Child Fetal Neonatal Ed. 2021;106:460–6.
62. Stensvold HJ, Strommen K, Lang AM, Abrahamsen TG, Steen EK, Pripp AH, Ronnestad AE. Early enhance parenteral nutrition, hyperglycemia, and death among extremely low-birthweight infants. JAMA Pediatr. 2015;169:1003–10.
63. Heimann K, Peschgens T, Kwiecien R, Stanzel S, Hoernchen H, Merz U. Are recurrent hyperglycemic episodes and median blood glucose level a prognostic factor for increased morbidity and mortality in premature infants </=1500 g? J Perinat Med. 2007;35:245–8.
64. Hays SP, Smith EO, Sunehag AL. Hyperglycemia is a risk factor for early death and morbidity in extremely low birth-weight infants. Pediatrics. 2006;118:1811–8.
65. Blanco CL, McGill-Vargas LL, McCurnin D, Quinn AR. Hyperglycemia increases the risk of death in extremely preterm baboons. Pediatr Res. 2013;73:337–43.
66. Tottman AC, Alsweiler JM, Bloomfield FH, Pan M, Harding JE. Relationship between measures of neonatal glycemia, neonatal illness, and 2-year outcomes in very preterm infants. J Pediatr. 2017;188:115–21.

67. Al-Mouqdad MM, Abdalgader AT, Abdelrahim A, Almosbahi FA, Khalil TM, Asfour YS, Asfour SS. Association of early dysglycemia with intraventricular hemorrhage and mortality in very low birth weight infants. Eur J Pediatr. 2024;183:5331–7.
68. Alsweiler JM, Harding JE, Bloomfield FH. Neonatal hyperglycaemia increases mortality and morbidity in preterm lambs. Neonatology. 2013;103:83–90.
69. Gonzalez Villamizar JD, Haapala JL, Scheurer JM, Rao R, Ramel SE. Relationships between early nutrition, illness, and later outcomes among infants born preterm with hyperglycemia. J Pediatr. 2020;223:29–33.e2.
70. Guleria RS, Pan J, Dipette D, Singh US. Hyperglycemia inhibits retinoic acid-induced activation of Rac1, prevents differentiation of cortical neurons, and causes oxidative stress in a rat model of diabetic pregnancy. Diabetes. 2006;55:3326–34.
71. Garvin J, Semenikhina M, Liu Q, Rarick K, Isaeva E, Levchenko V, Staruschenko A, Palygin O, Harder D, Cohen S. Astrocytic responses to high glucose impair barrier formation in cerebral microvessel endothelial cells. Am J Physiol Regul Integr Comp Physiol. 2022;322:R571–80.
72. Scheurer J, Gray H, Demerath E, Rao R, Ramel S. Diminished growth and lower adiposity in hyperglycemic very low birth weight neonates at 4 months corrected age. J Perinatol. 2016;36:145–50.
73. Ramel SE, Long JD, Gray H, Durrwachter-Erno K, Demerath EW, Rao R. Neonatal hyperglycemia and diminished long-term growth in very low birth weight preterm infants. J Perinatol. 2013;33:882–6.
74. Wang J, Yue X, Meng C, Wang Z, Jin X, Cui X, Yang J, Shan C, Gao Z, Yang Y, Li J, Chang B, Chang B. Acute hyperglycemia may induce renal tubular injury through mitophagy inhibition. Front Endocrinol (Lausanne). 2020;11:536213.
75. Crump C, Winkleby MA, Sundquist K, Sundquist J. Risk of diabetes among young adults born preterm in Sweden. Diabetes Care. 2011;34:1109–13.
76. Hofman PL, Regan F, Jackson WE, Jefferies C, Knight DB, Robinson EM, Cutfield WS. Premature birth and later insulin resistance. N Engl J Med. 2004;351:2179–86.
77. Barco VS, Gallego FQ, Miranda CA, Souza MR, Volpato GT, Damasceno DC. Hyperglycemia influences the cell proliferation and death of the rat endocrine pancreas in the neonatal period. Life Sci. 2024;351:122854.
78. Bansal A, Bloomfield FH, Connor KL, Dragunow M, Thorstensen EB, Oliver MH, Sloboda DM, Harding JE, Alsweiler JM. Glucocorticoid-induced preterm birth and neonatal hyperglycemia alter ovine beta-cell development. Endocrinology. 2015;156:3763–76.
79. Dani C, Luzzati M, Corsini I, Poggi C, Vangi V, Coviello C, Pratesi S. Cardiac hypertrophy associated with insulin therapy in extremely preterm infants. Paediatr Drugs. 2023;25:453–7.
80. Alsweiler JM, Harding JE, Bloomfield FH. Tight glycemic control with insulin in hyperglycemic preterm babies: a randomized controlled trial. Pediatrics. 2012;129:639–47.
81. Zamir I, Stoltz Sjöström E, Edstedt Bonamy A-K, Mohlkert L-A, Norman M, Domellöf M. Postnatal nutritional intakes and hyperglycemia as determinants of blood pressure at 6.5 years of age in children born extremely preterm. Pediatr Res. 2019;86:115–21.
82. Hamayun J, Mohlkert LA, Stoltz Sjostrom E, Domellof M, Norman M, Zamir I. Association between neonatal intakes and hyperglycemia, and left heart and aortic dimensions at 6.5 years of age in children born extremely preterm. J Clin Med. 2021;10:2554.
83. McClure Yauch L, Ennis-Czerniak K, Frey Ii WH, Tkac I, Rao RB. Intranasal insulin attenuates the long-term adverse effects of neonatal hyperglycemia on the hippocampus in rats. Dev Neurosci. 2022;44:590–602.
84. Guiducci S, Meggiolaro L, Righetto A, Piccoli M, Baraldi E, Galderisi A. Neonatal hyperglycemia and neurodevelopmental outcomes in preterm infants: a review. Children (Basel). 2022;9:1541
85. van der Lugt NM, Smits-Wintjens VE, van Zwieten PH, Walther FJ. Short and long term outcome of neonatal hyperglycemia in very preterm infants: a retrospective follow-up study. BMC Pediatr. 2010;10:52.

Chapter 11
Prophylactic and Treatment Approaches to Prevent and Treat Neonatal Hyperglycemia

Jane Alsweiler and Jane Harding

Introduction

As noted by Paulsen and colleagues, "Current evidence of long-term health outcomes following early hyperglycemia in VLBW infants does not provide high-quality recommendations to guide assessment and treatment of early hyperglycemia." [1] Well-designed, large randomized controlled trials and prospective studies are needed to determine which neonates are at risk for long-term metabolic and neurodevelopmental compromise after hyperglycemia, glucose concentration thresholds above which neurodevelopmental outcomes are impaired, the duration of different high glucose concentrations that definitively increase the risk of adverse metabolic and neurodevelopmental outcomes, and what interventions can prevent or at least decrease the risk of long-term adverse outcomes that compromise normal later life metabolism, neurodevelopment, cognition, and behavior. "Prospective studies using standardized approaches to early nutrition, evaluation and treatment of hyperglycemia, and outcome assessment will improve the quality of evidence to inform clinical practice for management of hyperglycemia" [1].

J. Alsweiler (✉)
Department of Paediatrics: Child and Youth Health, School of Medicine, University of Auckland, Auckland, New Zealand
e-mail: j.alsweiler@auckland.ac.nz

J. Harding
Liggins Institute, University of Auckland, Auckland, New Zealand

D. H. Adamkin, W. W. Hay, Jr. (eds.), *Disorders of Neonatal Glycemia*,
https://doi.org/10.1007/978-3-032-29094-6_11

Prophylactic and Treatment Approaches to Prevent and Treat Neonatal Hyperglycemia

Prevention

As extreme prematurity is the primary cause of neonatal hyperglycemia, preventing preterm birth would be the most effective strategy to prevent neonatal hyperglycemia. However, global rates of preterm birth have remained stable over the past decade and are unlikely to decline significantly in the near future (Fig. 11.1) [2].

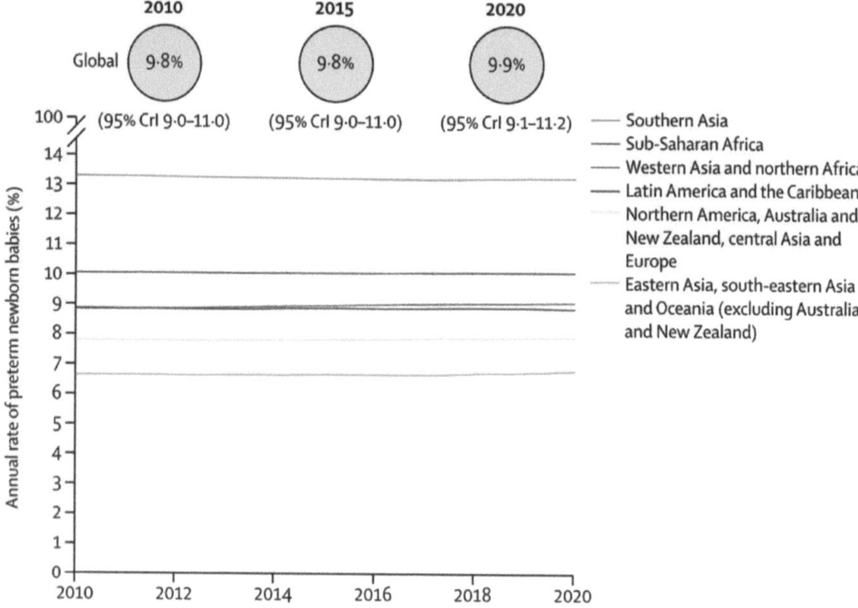

Fig. 11.1 Regional and worldwide trends in preterm birth between 2010 and 2020. (From: Ohuma et al. [2])

Alternative Potential Strategies to Reduce the Incidence of Neonatal Hyperglycemia Include Changes to Nutrition, Monitoring, and Drug Treatments

Nutrition

Several nutritional factors contribute to hyperglycemia, including high glucose load, low protein intake, and delayed transition to enteral feeding. Therefore, changes to nutritional support offered to very preterm babies offer a potential strategy to reduce the incidence of neonatal hyperglycemia.

A recent trial of early additional protein in extremely preterm babies did not report the incidence of hyperglycemia, but there was no difference in mortality or morbidities commonly associated with neonatal hyperglycemia, such as retinopathy of prematurity, intraventricular hemorrhage or sepsis [3]. However, in the babies who received additional protein there was an increase in refeeding syndrome, defined as serum phosphate concentration of <1.4 mmol/L and serum calcium concentration of >2.8 mmol/L on day 5 after birth. Refeeding syndrome is a known complication of malnutrition treated with enteral or intravenous refeeding, which in adults and children may cause a potentially fatal cluster of fluid and electrolyte disturbances, including hyperglycemia (Fig. 11.2).

Preterm birth, especially of growth restricted babies, may be described as a state of malnutrition, which is routinely treated with intravenous refeeding, potentially increasing the risk of refeeding syndrome in babies born preterm. Refeeding syndrome in extremely low birthweight preterm babies is associated with an increase in morbidity, including intraventricular haemorrhage, and mortality [4]. Low phosphate concentrations, one of the diagnostic features of refeeding syndrome, has been associated with an increased risk of hyperglycemia in preterm babies [5]. It is possible that supplementing the nutrition of very preterm babies with additional phosphate could reduce the incidence of refeeding syndrome, including hyperglycemia and associated morbidities, but there is currently no evidence available.

An additional strategy to reduce the incidence of neonatal hyperglycemia may be a reduction of the amount of intravenous dextrose given to preterm babies. Observational data of very low birth weight preterm babies has shown that babies who received more protein, less fat, and less carbohydrate, had lower mean blood glucose concentrations (BGC) and less hyperglycemia [6]. However, a potential concern about reducing glucose in very preterm babies is that it could increase the risk of hypoglycemia, which may impair brain development, and reduce calorie intake and therefore growth. There have been several randomized trials that have randomized babies to restricted amounts of fluid which, as the concentration of dextrose in the fluid was not altered, also meant they received less dextrose [7]. In the earliest and largest trial, preterm babies randomized to less parenteral fluid received less calories, had more dehydration and lost more weight than babies who received more parenteral fluid, but also had a lower incidence of patent ductus arteriosus and necrotizing enterocolitis [8]. ESPGHAN guidelines give guidance on the amount of glucose preterm babies should receive to enable growth and energy to the

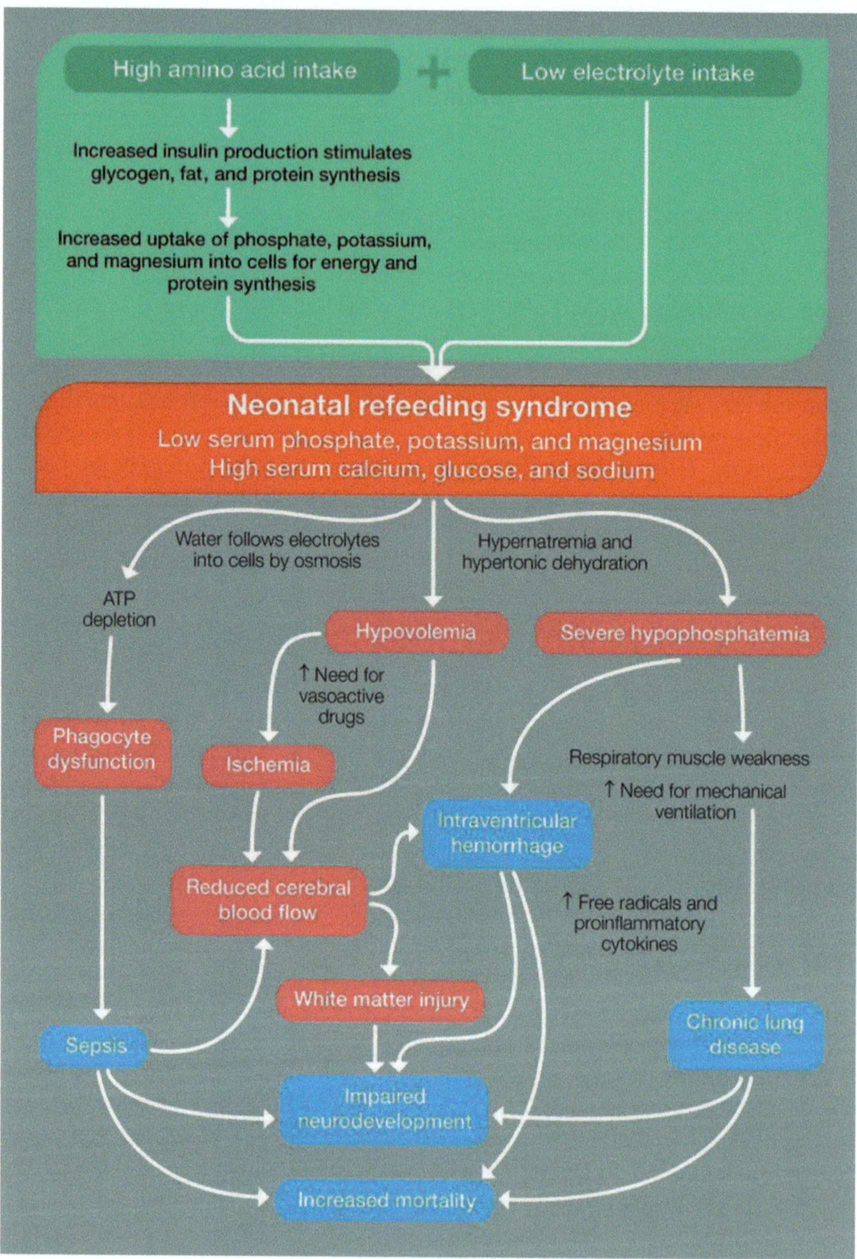

Fig. 11.2 Mechanisms involved in neonatal refeeding syndrome. (From: Cormack et al. [4])

brain [9]. It is recommended to titrate the glucose infusion rate based on the BGC prior to starting insulin treatment, although there is little evidence to support this practice.

There is observational evidence that the longer it takes to transition to enteral feeds from parenteral nutrition, the greater the risk of developing hyperglycemia [6]. While rapid transition to enteral feeds is associated with an increased risk of necrotizing enterocolitis in observational studies [10], a large randomized controlled trial has shown that rates of increased enteral feeding up to 30 mg/kg/day are safe [11]. Although the trial did not report on the incidence of hyperglycemia, it would be considered good practice to transition preterm babies to enteral feeds at a rate of 30 mg/kg/day.

Low concentrations of Insulin-like growth factor 1 (IGF-1) in preterm babies are associated with neonatal hyperglycemia [12]. It has been proposed that IGF-1 supplementation may improve insulin sensitivity, which could theoretically reduce hyperglycemia [13]. A trial of recombinant human insulin-like growth factor 1 complexed with its binding protein (rhIGF1/rhIGFBP-3) supplementation in extremely preterm neonates found that rhIGF-1/rhIGFBP-3 did not decrease retinopathy of prematurity severity or retinopathy of prematurity occurrence, although it did reduce the incidence of bronchopulmonary dysplasia, but did not report on the incidence of hyperglycemia [14]. The potential impact of IGF-1 therapy on glycemic control remains unexplored in randomized trials.

Continuous Glucose Monitoring

Newer technologies, such as continuous glucose monitoring (CGM) and computerised treatment algorithms offer a new approach to preventing neonatal hyperglycemia. CGM is well tolerated in even extremely low birth weight preterm babies [15]. Interstitial glucose results from CGM correlate well with point of care devices with minimal bias, (Fig. 11.3) and provide more detailed continuous data. Therefore, although single readings may not be accurate, the device can help to detect periods of both hyperglycemia and hypoglycemia.

A randomized controlled trial of very-low-birth-weight preterm babies randomized to have real time continuous glucose monitoring or masked continuous glucose monitoring found that babies in the real time CGM group received more intravenous glucose than the masked CGM group, but had a lower mean interstitial glucose concentration (glucose concentration 6.5 mmol/L v 7 mmol/L), with no difference between the time the groups spent in the hypoglycemia or hyperglycemia (>15 mmol/L) range or in the amount of insulin they received [16]. The proportion of time sensor glucose concentration between 2.6 and 10 mmol/L in the first week after birth was greater in the real time CGM group. CGM has also been shown to reduce the number of dysglycemic episodes (interstitial glucose concentration <2.6 mmol/L or >10 mmol/L) when alarms are set at a tighter level (3.4 mmol/L and 7.8 mmol/L) compared to standard values (2.61 mmol/L and 10 mmol/L), and a

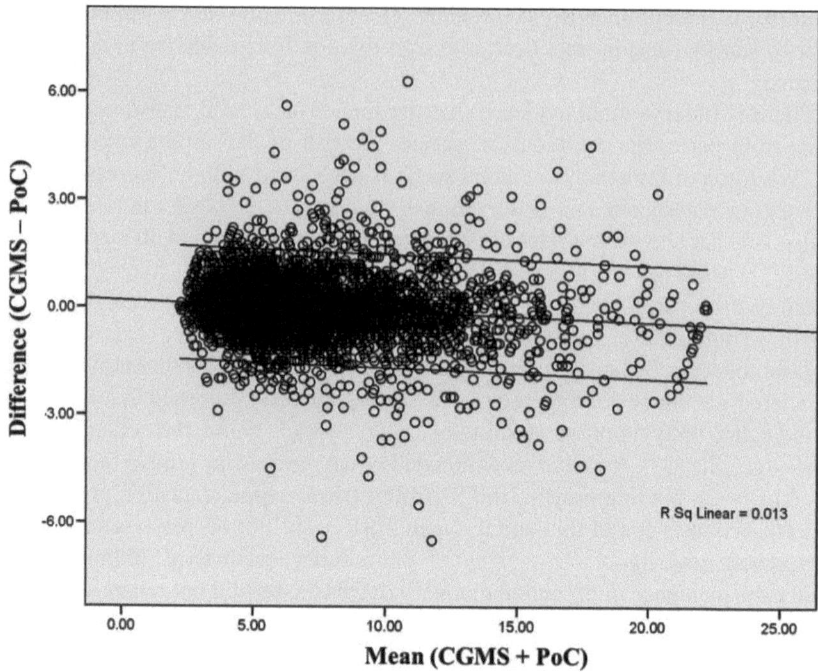

Fig. 11.3 CGM v point of care glucose (mmol/L) testing Bland Altman plot. Horizontal axis represents the mean of the sensor and point of care glucose measurement. Vertical axis represents the difference between the sensor and point of care glucose measure. (From: Beardsall et al. [15])

glucose infusion rate of 33% glucose titrated to maintaining the interstitial glucose concentration between the alarm limits [17]. Closed-loop insulin delivery combining CGM, algorithmic control, and insulin infusion can also dramatically improve time spent in target glucose range in extremely preterm infants (Fig. 11.3). This 'artificial pancreas'–style approach appears safe and feasible, though its impact on clinical outcomes remains to be evaluated in larger trials [18] (Fig. 11.4).

Prophylactic Insulin

As neonatal hyperglycemia is at least in part due to insulin deficiency, it is possible that preventing babies developing hyperglycemia with early insulin treatment to maintain euglycemia may improve outcomes [19]. The NIRTURE trial was a multicentre randomized controlled trial of very low birth weight infants, who were randomized to receive insulin (0.05 U/kg/h) with variable dextrose support to maintain euglycemia (BGC 4–8 mmol/L) from 24 h after birth until 7 days after birth or standard management, with a primary outcome of mortality [20]. The trial randomized 389 babies, all of whom had continuous glucose monitoring, before the trial

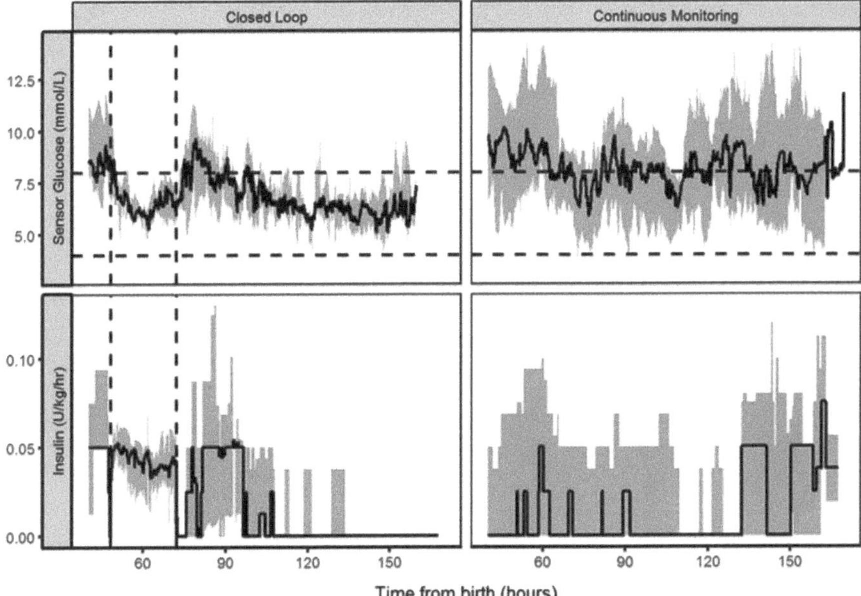

Fig. 11.4 Glucose control and insulin delivery median (IQR) of sensor glucose and insulin infused in babies randomized to closed-loop management or continuous glucose monitoring with paper algorithm (control). The closed-loop intervention period is denoted by the vertical lines, and the target glucose range 4.0–8.0 mmol/L is denoted by horizontal lines. (From: Beardsall et al. [18])

was suspended before reaching the planned sample size based on a combination of futility associated with the primary outcome and concern about potential harm. The babies randomized to the intervention had lower mean interstitial glucose concentrations, less hyperglycemia, more hypoglycemia, and received more carbohydrate (Fig. 11.5). More babies who received the intervention died prior to day 28, with no statistical difference in the proportion of babies who died before the expected date of delivery. Therefore, although prophylactic treatment with insulin in babies at risk of neonatal hyperglycemia did reduce hyperglycemia, there were increased risks of hypoglycemia and mortality, and this practice is not recommended.

Preventing neonatal hyperglycemia remains a complex challenge, tightly linked to the physiology of extreme preterm birth. Nutritional interventions, such as optimizing macronutrient composition and reducing glucose load, show promise but require careful balancing to avoid hypoglycemia and growth restriction. Transitioning preterm babies to enteral feeds swiftly, within the known thresholds of safety [11], may help to reduce the incidence of hyperglycemia.

Emerging concepts such refeeding syndrome and IGF-1 deficiency offer interesting mechanistic insights but yet lack interventional evidence. Real-time CGM monitoring and computer algorithms show promise as strategies to improve glucose homeostasis in extremely preterm babies. Prophylactic insulin therapy, though effective in lowering glucose concentrations, carries unacceptable risks and is not

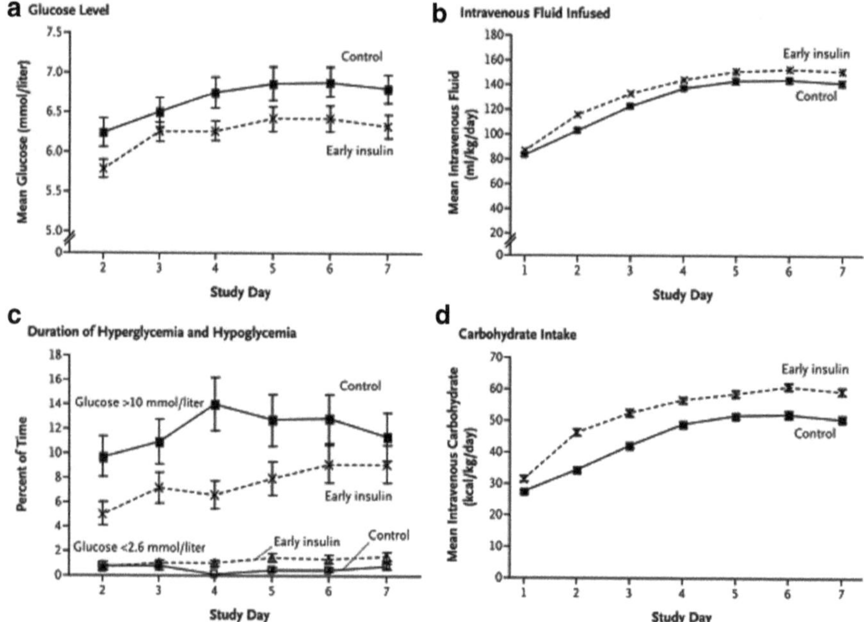

Fig. 11.5 Efficacy outcomes of early insulin therapy. (**a**) Glucose Level; (**b**) Intravenous Fluid Infused; (**c**) Duration of Hyperglycemia and Hypoglycemia; (**d**) Carbohydrate Intake. (From: Beardsall et al. [20])

recommended. Further research is needed to identify safe and effective strategies that reduce hyperglycemia without compromising neurodevelopment or survival.

Treatment of Neonatal Hyperglycemia

The primary goals of treatment are to maintain blood glucose concentrations (BGC) within a safe range, avoiding both hypoglycemia and prolonged hyperglycemia, and to reduce associated morbidities and mortality. Despite its prevalence, there is limited high-quality evidence guiding the safest and most effective treatment strategies for neonatal hyperglycemia.

Watchful Tolerance

An initial management strategy is often to tolerate higher blood glucose concentrations and not aggressively treat mild hyperglycemia. While higher blood glucose concentrations are associated with higher morbidity and mortality [21, 22], treatment of hyperglycemia, especially with insulin, carries the risk of neonatal

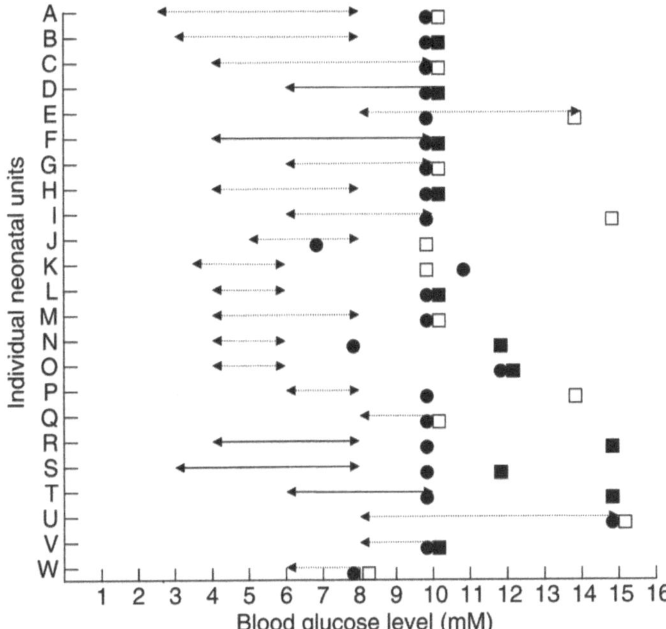

Fig. 11.6 Insulin use in premature hyperglycemic infants in the neonatal intensive care unit. (From: Alsweiler et al. [28])

hypoglycemia [23, 24]. Neonatal hypoglycemia is associated with brain injury, including the risk of seizures, long-term changes on MRI and neurodevelopmental impairment [25, 26]. In the absence of robust evidence supporting insulin's safety and long-term efficacy, watchful tolerance may be appropriate for mild or short-lived hyperglycemia. However, severe or prolonged hyperglycemia is associated with mortality and significant morbidity [22, 27], therefore it is standard practice to treat neonatal hyperglycemia, although there is substantial variation in clinical practice on the thresholds at which treatment is begun (Fig. 11.6) [24, 28, 29].

Furthermore, the use of insulin for neonatal hyperglycemia has reduced over time (Fig. 11.7) [28].

Reduction of Dextrose

The second management option is to reduce the amount of glucose the baby receives by reducing the dextrose infusion concentration and/or volume. The ESPGHAN guidelines recommend that hyperglycemia >8 mmol/L (145 mg/dL) should be avoided in neonatal ICU patients because it is associated with increased morbidity and mortality, and that insulin treatment should be started for BGC consistently about 10 mmol/L if reasonable adaptation of glucose infusion rate has

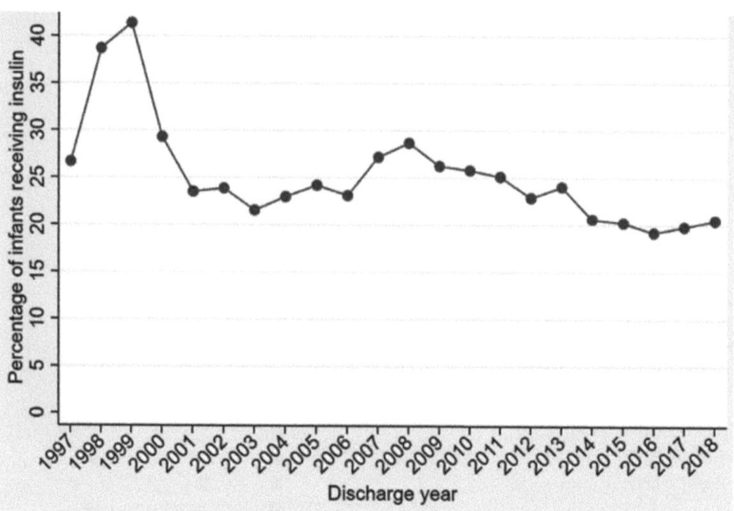

Fig. 11.7 Decline in the percentage of infants receiving insulin over time. (From: Titchiner et al. [24])

been insufficient [9]. This implies that for babies with a BGC of >8 mmol/L, the recommendation is to reduce the glucose infusion rate. ESPGHAN suggests starting the glucose infusion rate at approximately 4–6 mg/kg/min on Day 1 and increasing to 8–10 mg/kg/min by Days 2–5, depending on tolerance and metabolic needs. If a baby with hyperglycemia is receiving a glucose infusion rate above these thresholds, reducing the glucose load may be warranted. When dextrose is being given as part of the parenteral nutrition infusion, care needs to be taken not to reduce the protein intake below recommended levels when reducing the dextrose load [30].

Insulin Treatment

Insulin is a lifesaving, standard-of-care treatment for children and adults with type 1 diabetes mellitus, a condition of absolute insulin deficiency, and a cornerstone of therapy in type 2 diabetes mellitus, which is characterized by insulin resistance and relative deficiency [31]. While hyperglycemia in preterm neonates arises from a combination of insulin deficiency and insulin insensitivity [32], suggesting that insulin therapy would be beneficial, there is limited high-quality evidence to guide the use of insulin in this population.

There is animal evidence that treatment with insulin in preterm lambs who had dextrose-overload induced hyperglycemia reduces the risk of mortality secondary to hyperglycemia, but insulin increases the risk of hypoglycemia and does not reverse the effects of hyperglycemia on growth [33].

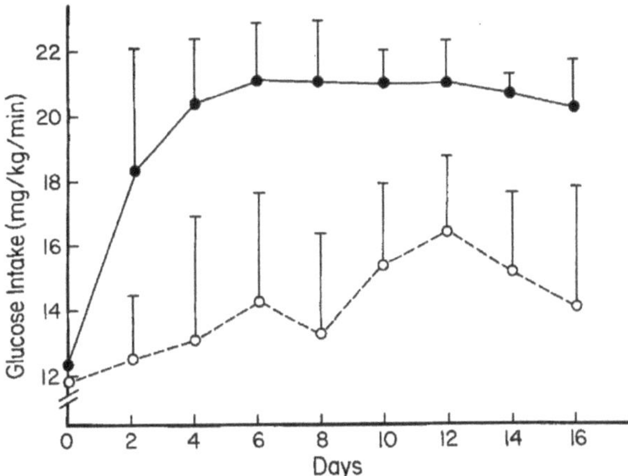

Fig. 11.8 Mean (+/− SD) glucose infusion rate per day (mg/kg/minute) in insulin-treated (solid line) and control (dashed line) infants. (From: Collins et al. [34])

However, there is little evidence on the use of insulin in preterm babies with neonatal hyperglycemia. The only randomized controlled trial of insulin compared with no insulin in hyperglycemic (BGC ≥ 10 mmol/L) preterm babies was done in ELBW babies with glycosuria and a nonprotein parenteral intake <120 kcal/kg/day. Eligible babies were randomized to intravenous insulin infusion aiming to keep the BGC 5.5–9.9 mmol/L or standard care, with a primary outcome of glucose tolerance [34]. Babies in the insulin group received more glucose than those in the standard care group, (Fig. 11.8) and gained more weight over the first 2 weeks after birth, with no difference in the incidence of hypoglycemia. However, this was a small trial of only 24 babies and was not powered to detect important clinical outcomes.

A systematic review and a meta-analysis of insulin treatment of neonatal hyperglycemia primarily comprised of observational studies [23]. The findings indicated that, after adjustment for known confounders, there was no statistically significant difference in outcomes between infants treated with insulin and those who were not. As expected, unadjusted data showed poorer outcomes in the insulin-treated group, likely due to greater baseline illness severity. A recent large population-based study also reported an association between insulin use and increased risk of death and retinopathy of prematurity, even after adjusting for gestational age; however, this may similarly reflect the more compromised clinical condition of infants receiving insulin [24].

Insulin is usually administered as a continuous intravenous infusion. While there are some initial cases that describe insulin being administered as a continuous subcutaneous infusion, further research is needed before this is introduced as a standard technique [35].

Tight glycemic control with insulin in preterm babies has been investigated by a randomized controlled trial [36]. In the HINT trial preterm babies (<1500 g or <30 weeks gestational age) with hyperglycemia (BGC > 8.5 mmol/L on two consecutive samples) were randomized to treatment with insulin to maintain the BGC at 4–6 mmol/L or 8–10 mmol/L, with a primary outcome of lower leg length growth rate. Babies randomized to tight glycemic control had slower lower leg growth, less glycosuria and a higher incidence of hypoglycemia. Long term follow-up of the children in this trial at 7 years of age, showed no difference in neurodevelopment between the two groups. However, tight glycemic control reduced height, increased height-adjusted lean mass, and reduced fasting blood glucose concentrations [37].

Conclusions

Treatment of neonatal hyperglycemia remains a balancing act between mitigating the risks of high glucose concentrations and avoiding the harms of overtreatment. Mild or transient hyperglycemia may not require intervention, especially given the risks of hypoglycemia and the lack of evidence supporting insulin's long-term benefits. Reducing glucose intake is a logical first step and aligns with current guidelines but must be done cautiously to avoid compromising energy supply and growth.

Insulin therapy may be necessary in cases of persistent or severe hyperglycemia but should be approached with caution. The limited trial data and observational evidence suggest no clear benefit, and potential harm.

Ultimately, the safest and most effective treatment strategy may depend on the infant's gestational age, clinical condition, nutritional status, and capacity for glucose regulation. Further research is urgently needed to define optimal thresholds, refine insulin protocols, and explore alternative therapies that support metabolic stability without increasing risk.

References

1. Paulsen ME, Brown SJ, Satrom KM, Scheurer JM, Ramel SE, Rao RB. Long-term outcomes after early neonatal hyperglycemia in VLBW infants: a systematic review. Neonatology. 2021;118:509–21.
2. Ohuma EO, Moller A-B, Bradley E, Chakwera S, Hussain-Alkhateeb L, Lewin A, et al. National, regional, and global estimates of preterm birth in 2020, with trends from 2010: a systematic analysis. Lancet. 2023;402:1261–71.
3. Bloomfield FH, Jiang Y, Harding JE, Crowther CA, Cormack BE. Early amino acids in extremely preterm infants and neurodisability at 2 years. N Engl Med J. 2022;387:1661–72.
4. Cormack BE, Jiang Y, Harding JE, Crowther CA, Bloomfield FH. Neonatal refeeding syndrome and clinical outcome in extremely low-birth-weight babies: secondary cohort analysis rrom the ProVIDe Trial. JPEN J Parenter Enteral Nutr. 2021;45:65–78.
5. Al-Wassia H, Lyon AW, Rose SM, Sauve RS, Fenton TR. Hypophosphatemia is prevalent among preterm infants less than 1,500 grams. Am J Perinatol. 2019;36:1412–9.
6. Tottman AC, Bloomfield FH, Cormack BE, Harding JE, Mohd Slim MA, Weston AF, Alsweiler JM. Relationships between early nutrition and blood glucose concentrations in very preterm infants. J Pediatr Gastroenterol Nutr. 2018;66:960–6.
7. Bell EF, Acarregui MJ. Restricted versus liberal water intake for preventing morbidity and mortality in preterm infants. Cochrane Database Syst Rev. 2000;(2):CD000503.

8. Bell EF, Warburton D, Stonestreet BS, Oh W. Effect of fluid administration on the development of symptomatic patent ductus arteriosus and congestive heart failure in premature infants. N Engl J Med. 1980;302:598–604.
9. Messoten D, Joosten K, Van Kempen A, Verbruggen S, the ESPGHAN/ESPEN/ESPR working group of pediatric parenteral nutrition. ESPGHAN/ESPEN/ESPR Guidelines on pediatric parenteral nutrition: carbohydrates. Clin Nutr. 2018;37:2337–43.
10. Henderson G, Craig S, Brocklehurst P, McGuire W. Enteral feeding regimens and necrotizing enterocolitis in preterm infants: a multicentre case-control study. Arch Dis Child Fetal Neonatal Ed. 2009;94:F120–3.
11. Dorling J, Abbott J, Berrington J, Bosiak B, Bowler U, Boyle E, Embleton N, Hewer O, Johnson S, Juszczak E, Leaf A, Linsell L, McCormick K, McGuire W, Omar O, Partlett C, Patel M, Roberts T, Stenson B, Townend J, SIFT Investigators Group. Controlled trial of two incremental milk-feeding rates in preterm infants. N Engl J Med. 2019;381:1434–43.
12. Beardsall K, Vanhaesebrouck S, Frystyk J, Ogilvy-Stuart AL, Vanhole C, van Weissenbruch M, Midgley P, Thio M, Cornette L, Gill B, Ossuetta I, Iglesias I, Theyskens C, de Jong M, Ahluwalia JS, de Zegher F, Dunger DB, NIRTURE Study Group. Relationship between insulin-like growth factor I levels, early insulin treatment, and clinical outcomes of very low birth weight infants. J Pediatr. 2014;164:1038–1044.e1.
13. Hellström A, Ley D, Hansen-Pupp I, Hallberg B, Löfqvist C, van Marter L, van Weissenbruch M, Ramenghi LA, Beardsall K, Dunger D, Hård AL, Smith LE. Insulin-like growth factor 1 has multisystem effects on foetal and preterm infant development. Acta Paediatr. 2016;105:576–86.
14. Ley D, Hallberg B, Hansen-Pupp I, Dani C, Ramenghi LA, Marlow N, Beardsall K, Bhatti F, Dunger D, Higginson JD, Mahaveer A, Mezu-Ndubuisi OJ, Reynolds P, Giannantonio C, van Weissenbruch M, Barton N, Tocoian A, Hamdani M, Jochim E, Mangili A, Chung JK, Turner MA, Smith LEH, Hellström A, Study team. rhIGF-1/rhIGFBP-3 in preterm infants: a phase 2 randomized controlled trial. J Pediatr. 2019;206:56–65 e8.
15. Beardsall K, Vanhaesebrouch S, Ogilvy-Stuart A, Vanhole C, Vanweissenbruch M, Midgely P. Validation of the continuous glucose monitoring sensor in preterm infants. Arch Dis Child Fetal Neonatal Ed. 2013;98:F136–40.
16. Beardsall K, Thomson L, Iglesias-Platas I, van Weissenbruch MM, Bond S, Dunger D. Continuous glucose monitoring in the neonatal intensive care unit: need for practical guidelines – authors' reply. Lancet Child Adolesc Health. 2021;5:e16.
17. Perri A, Tiberi E, Giordano L, Sbordone A, Patti ML, Iannotta R, et al. Strict glycemic control in very low birthweight infants using a continuous glucose monitoring system: a randomized controlled trial. Arch Dis Child Fetal Neonatal Ed. 2022;107:26–31.
18. Beardsall K, Thomson L, Elleri D, Dunger DB, Hovorka R. Feasibility of automated insulin delivery guided by continuous glucose monitoring in preterm infants. Arch Dis Child Fetal Neonatal Ed. 2020;105:279–84.
19. Salis ER, Reith DM, Wheeler BJ, Broadbent RS, Medlicott NJ. Hyperglycemic preterm neonates exhibit insulin resistance and low insulin production. BMJ Paediatr. 2017;1:e000160.
20. Beardsall K, Vanhaesebrouck S, Ogilvy-Stuart AL, Vanhole C, Palmer CR, van Weissenbruch M, Midgley P, Thompson M, Thio M, Cornette L, Ossuetta I, Iglesias I, Theyskens C, de Jong M, Ahluwalia JS, de Zegher F, Dunger DB. Early insulin therapy in very-low-birth-weight infants. N Engl J Med. 2008;359(18):1873–84.
21. Zamir I, Tornevi A, Abrahamsson T, Ahlsson F, Engström E, Hallberg B, Hansen-Pupp I, Sjöström ES, Domellöf M. Hyperglycemia in extremely preterm infants-insulin treatment, mortality and nutrient intakes. J Pediatr. 2018;200:104–110.e1.
22. Rath CP, Shivamallappa M, Muthusamy S, Rao SC, Patole S. Outcomes of very preterm infants with neonatal hyperglycemia: a systematic review and meta-analysis. Arch Dis Child Fetal Neonatal Ed. 2022;107:1–12.
23. Patidar N, Rath CP, Rao S, Patole S. Outcomes of very preterm infants with hyperglycemia treated with insulin: a systematic review and meta-analysis. Acta Paediatr. 2023;112:1157–64.
24. Titchiner D, Hornik C, Benjamin R, Tolia V, Smith PB, Greenberg RG. Insulin for treatment of neonatal hyperglycemia in premature infants: prevalence over time and association with outcomes. Am J Perinatol. 2024;41:e1008–14.

25. Edwards T, Alsweiler JM, Gamble GD, Griffith R, Lin L, McKinlay CJD, Rogers JA, Thompson B, Wouldes TA, Harding JE. Neurocognitive outcomes at age 2 years after neonatal hypoglycemia in a cohort of participants from the hPOD randomized trial. JAMA Netw Open. 2022;5:e2235989.
26. Nivins S, Kennedy E, Thompson B, Gamble GD, Alsweiler JM, Metcalfe R, McKinlay CJD, Harding JE, Children with Hypoglycemia and their Later Development Study Group. Associations between neonatal hypoglycemia and brain volumes, cortical thickness and white matter microstructure in mid-childhood: an MRI study. NeuroImage Clin. 2022;33:102943.
27. Zhu J, He X, Guo M. Association of early hyperglycemia with morbidity and mortality in very low birth weight infants. BMC Pediatr. 2025;25:667.
28. Alsweiler JM, Kuschel CA, Bloomfield FH. Survey of the management of neonatal hyperglycemia in Australasia. J Paediatr Child Health. 2007;43:632–5.
29. Frithiof LH, Domellöf M, Zamir IN. Management of neonatal hyperglycemia in Sweden—a survey study. Acta Paediatr. 2025;114:1399–404.
30. Cormack BE, Bloomfield FH. Increased protein intake decreases postnatal growth faltering in ELBW babies. Arch Dis Child Fetal Neonatal Ed. 2013;98:F399–404.
31. Tegegne BA, Adugna A, Yenet A, Yihunie Belay W, Yibeltal Y, Dagne A, Hibstu Teffera Z, Amare GA, Abebaw D, Tewabe H, Abebe RB, Zeleke TK. A critical review on diabetes mellitus type 1 and type 2 management approaches: from lifestyle modification to current and novel targets and therapeutic agents. Front Endocrinol (Lausanne). 2024;15:1440456.
32. Blanco C, Liang H, Joya-Galeana J, DeFronzo R, McCurnin D, Musi N. The ontogeny of insulin signaling in the preterm baboon model. Endocrinology. 2010;151(5):1990–7.
33. Alsweiler JM, Harding JE, Bloomfield F. Neonatal hyperglycemia increases mortality and morbidity in preterm lambs. Neonatology. 2013;103:83–90.
34. Collins JWJ, Hoppe M, Brown K, Edidin DV, Padbury J, Ogata ES. A controlled trial of insulin infusion and parenteral nutrition in extremely low birth weight infants with glucose intolerance. J Pediatr. 1991;118:921–7.
35. Böettger M, Zhou T, Knopp J, Chase JG, Heep A, von Vangerow M, Cloppenburg E, Lange M. Treatment of severe hyperglycemia in extremely preterm infants using continuous subcutaneous insulin therapy. J Clin Res Pediatr Endocrinol. 2024;164:443–9.
36. Alsweiler JM, Harding JE, Bloomfield FH. Tight glycemic control with insulin in hyperglycemic preterm babies: a randomized controlled trial. Pediatrics. 2012;129:639–47.
37. Tottman AC, Alsweiler JM, Bloomfield FH, Gamble G, Jiang Y, Leung M, Poppe T, Thompson B, Wouldes TA, Harding JE, PIANO Study Group. Long-term outcomes of hyperglycemic preterm infants randomized to tight glycemic control. J Pediatr. 2018;193:68–75.

Index

D. H. Adamkin, W. W. Hay. Jr. (eds.), *Disorders of Neonatal Glycemia*,
https://doi.org/10.1007/978-3-032-29094-6

E

F

G

H

O

P

R

S

T

V

Z

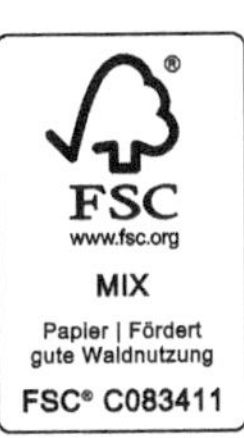

Zeitfracht Medien GmbH
Ferdinand-Jühlke-Straße 7
99095 Erfurt, Deutschland
produktsicherheit@kolibri360.de